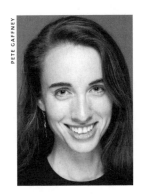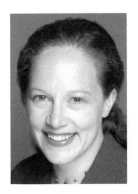

MIRANDA HAWKINS and SARAH KNOX are midwifery advocates who have had the benefit of midwifery care through miscarriages, complications and birth. They have been involved with the midwifery community for years, from helping to choose new students for the Midwifery Education Program at Ryerson University, to participating in policy issues, to establishing a client council for Toronto's largest midwifery practice. Miranda Hawkins is a writer who specializes in health issues. Sarah Knox is currently completing a Master's degree, with an emphasis on midwifery and education. Both women live in Toronto.

VICKI VAN WAGNER is a practising midwife and associate professor for the Midwifery Education Program at Ryerson University. She is internationally recognized as one of the architects of Ontario's midwifery legislation and a founder of the first university education program for midwives in Canada.

# The Midwifery Option

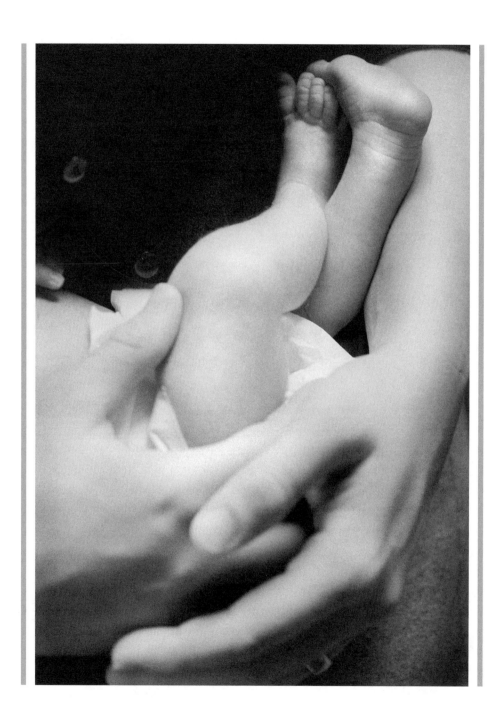

Sarah Knox and Miranda Hawkins

# THE MIDWIFERY OPTION

A Canadian Guide to the Birth Experience

HarperCollins*Publishers*Ltd

www.harpercanada.com

HarperCollins books may be purchased for educational, business, or sales
promotional use. For information please write: Special Markets Department,
HarperCollins Canada, 2 Bloor Street East, 20th Floor, Toronto, Ontario,
Canada M4W 1A8

First edition

National Library of Canada Cataloguing in Publication

Hawkins, Miranda
The midwifery option : a Canadian guide to the birth experience /
Miranda Hawkins and Sarah Knox.

Includes index.
ISBN 0-00-639425-6

1. Midwifery – Canada.  I. Knox, Sarah  II. Title.

RG950.H37 2003     618.2'0233'0971     C2002-904682-3

KRO 9 8 7 6 5 4 3 2 1

Printed and bound in Canada
Set in FF Quadraat

To the people who make me proud to be a mother:
Evangeline and Beatrice Freedman
Sandra and Bill Hawkins

MCH


I dedicate this to
Pete, Brazil and Esker
with love

SAK

# Contents

# Acknowledgements

Many people contributed to the making of this book, some providing inspiration and opinion, and others offering much needed backup while we juggled our lives, kids and this project. Thank you to everyone.

Tara Parker, Kristen Gill, Barb Strang, Hilary Knox, Carol Phillips and Karen Sabourin helped us shape the idea for this book by acting as a focus group at the outset of the project. Midwives all over the country contributed their time in interviews by phone and in person, and women and men offered us their stories and their personal perceptions of midwifery care. Other individuals graciously allowed us to photograph them, often on short notice. Whether or not a contribution ended up on these pages, the enthusiasm and passion that everyone shared with us is here. This book wouldn't exist without all of their offerings.

Pete Gaffney is responsible for all the beautiful images in this book and for keeping us laughing into the lens. Jenn Tiberio was very generous with her time and creativity in preparing the cover art for our proposal. Jenn McTaggart gave us invaluable feedback on the road to putting the proposal together. Teresa Pitman was instrumental in getting this book published. Debbie Burke-Benn gave us a much needed perspective in the final days of assembling the project.

Across the country, people took pity on us as we embarked on research trips on a shoestring budget. Katherine Side in Halifax provided room and board, and Catherine Berry was a great chauffeur and champion. The Wersehelers in Winnipeg, Barb Scriver in Edmonton, Kate Wadsworth in Calgary, Deirdre Byrne in Vancouver, the Coles in Victoria and Shannon Keenlyside in Montreal all provided space, sustenance and transportation. Everyone was very generous and it was great to make new friends.

Hilary Knox, Janine Dodge, Kate Harrison and Katrina Kilroy read numerous versions of the manuscript, providing comments, raising questions and offering encouragement. Vicki van Wagner and Dr. Michael Klein served as exacting and relentless editors, demanding accuracy, perspective and our very best work. Our editor at HarperCollins, Nicole Langlois, did us the great service of understanding what we were trying to accomplish from the moment we began, and making sure that we arrived there in the end.

We would never have set out on this journey without the wonderful care of our own midwives: Vicki van Wagner, Joyce Coombs, Katrina Kilroy, Elizabeth Allemang, Julie Corey, Merryn Tate, Sylvie Lemay and Pilar Chapman.

Lastly, and most importantly, our families and friends came through again and again on this project, as they do on everything. Sarah wishes to thank Hilary Knox for her substantial support since the moment this project was conceived. Many friends and family members offered support and contributions, in particular Phoebe Miles, and all of the Kinder Garden co-operative. Sarah could not have completed this project without her family who gave so much of themselves: Pete Gaffney, Brazil and Esker Gaffney-Knox. Miranda could not have written this book, or lived through her life in the past couple of years, without Evangeline and Beatrice Freedman, Sandra and Bill Hawkins, Alexa Dodge, Laurie Monsebraaten and Jeff Keay. Our love to you all.

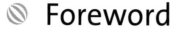 # Foreword

Vicki Van Wagner, RM

As a practising midwife and an educator, I have had the privilege of meeting many women and families who have told me that their experiences of childbirth with midwives made an important difference in their lives. Over more than twenty years as a midwife working in Toronto, and more recently in Nunavik, the Inuit region of northern Quebec, I have been present at the births of well over a thousand babies. I also teach midwifery students at the Midwifery Education Program at Ryerson University in Toronto, and in the Innulitsivik Health Centre in Puvrinituq and Inukjuak. Like many midwives, I am often asked to explain what I do, and have often wished for a resource like *The Midwifery Option*.

Two of the women for whom midwifery made a difference are Miranda Hawkins and Sarah Knox. I first met Miranda and Sarah as pregnant women receiving midwifery care in the practice where I work in central Toronto. After several babies and years of growing involvement with supporting the work of midwives, these two women met each other. Not only were they inspired by their pregnancy and birth experiences with midwives, they really wanted to do something to share their enthusiasm.

Their inspiration led them along several paths. They began organizing midwifery "clients" to create support systems and networks for each other in pregnancy and in the months of new parenthood. Like many midwifery advocates before them, they also worked at the policy and political level, in meetings and on committees, participating as partners with health professionals and policy makers as the relatively "new" profession of midwifery takes shape. Their work comes out of a long and very successful tradition in Canada of "consumer" and women's health activism for midwifery care.

As they became increasingly immersed in discussions with pregnant and postpartum women and their partners, and with midwives, Miranda and Sarah realized there was a need for more information about what midwifery care could be like for women and their families. They found that there was no English language book about midwifery in a current Canadian context. They decided they needed to write a book that would focus on why pregnant women and their partners choose midwifery care, on how midwives work and what the birth experience with midwives is like. This decision led to a journey that covered nine of the provinces and territories, talking with midwives, pregnant women in the care of midwives, and parents who had used midwifery care.

This is a book about midwifery, by midwifery clients, for those women and families who want to learn more about the care provided by midwives in Canada. *The Midwifery Option* combines "how to" information, consumer advocacy, history, politics and stories. Stories run throughout the text: stories of women in labour, parents with new babies, stories of births that could be seen as typical of midwifery care and of stories of very different kinds of births.

As the stories reveal, the pregnancy, birth and postpartum experiences that inspired this work were not always romantic or straightforward. This is significant, since an understanding of pregnancy and birth in all their potential complexity and contradiction are the cornerstones of *The Midwifery Option*. Miranda and Sarah's goal is to support the work that midwives do: to help women become actively involved in their health care during this potentially rewarding, but often challenging, and certainly changing, time of their lives.

Although it is a book about midwifery, *The Midwifery Option* is very different than a book written by a midwife or any other health professional. It does not attempt to describe the birth stories from a caregiver's perspective. It portrays birth with midwives through the eyes of the labouring woman, a parent in the first days postpartum and the mother invited to support another woman in labour. It is a book written by midwifery activists who want to share the inspiration they found in their birth process. It keeps the parents' perspectives and interests front and centre.

This focus on the experiential rather than the clinical does not mean this book should be passed over by clinicians as simply another "how to" book for the public. *The Midwifery Option* is a valuable book for clinicians as well. Its experiential perspective is the source of its relevance for midwives and other health professionals—as with midwifery care itself, it starts "with woman." Having the opportunity to look at the birth experience from the perspective of the parent is invaluable for health care providers working in the area of maternity care.

As Miranda and Sarah point out, there are many whose stories are not here, for instance, those who do not yet have access to midwifery, or those who cannot tell their stories due to language barriers. But what is clear from these stories is that women bring diverse needs and create very different kinds of meanings out of their childbearing experiences. This book may create opportunities for midwifery to grow and flourish in new places, and make space for more childbearing women to tell their stories.

*The Midwifery Option* reflects Canadian midwifery at an important moment in history. It is a time of turmoil and change in the health care system in general, and specifically in maternity care. Restructuring and reform have rocked many health care services. The ongoing development of "high tech" medicine and an increasing emphasis on genetics continue to transform childbearing. Midwifery is a small part of a very large and tumultuous system in Canada, but it occupies an interesting place as policy analysts predict a shortage of obstetric care providers in the next few decades. As an increasing number of small hospitals discontinue their obstetric services, there is a crisis in rural maternity care. Women from remote communities, especially in the north, continue to be evacuated to southern hospitals to give birth. And there is an immediate shortage of nurses internationally. Under these circumstances, childbirth as a family and community event is at risk and midwifery is under pressure to respond not only to the needs of individual clients, but to the needs of the system as a whole.

There is also a climate of change within the profession, as midwifery in Canada is in various stages of transition from unregulated to regulated practice. It has been less than a decade since midwifery was first recognized legally and integrated into Ontario's health care system, and in some provinces the process is still at the discussion stage. The profession is small and still growing into its role in the face of many demands.

This book reflects some of the many ways that midwifery is organized in different practices and provinces, but the variety of ways in which midwifery will evolve have only begun to be explored. There is both excitement and trepidation as the pressures from within and outside of midwifery means that midwifery is being defined and redefined as we speak.

Over the past two decades, as midwifery has become recognized and integrated into numerous provinces' health care systems, some midwifery advocates have worried about a decline of consumer involvement and activism. Miranda and Sarah's book is a sign that the passion about birth and midwifery, which led to the recognition of the profession of midwifery in Canada, is alive and well.

Vicki Van Wagner, RM
*Associate Professor,*
*Ryerson University Midwifery Education Program*
*Toronto, Ontario, Canada*

# Introduction

When you're pregnant, you can feel as if you're on display. People like to look at you. They like to come really close and touch your stomach. And they love to ask questions, such as "When are you due?" "Do you know whether you're having a girl or a boy?" "Got any names picked out?" But when you tell people you're having your baby without a doctor, that instead you've chosen a midwife, prepare yourself.

Many people can't shake the notion that midwives are remnants from the distant past. They're sure that all women who use midwives believe in the benefits of raw food, the evils of technology and the right to wear comfortable sandals—with socks.

Sure, today's midwifery client might be a yoga instructor from British Columbia. But she might just as well be a research analyst in Calgary, a Mennonite in Waterloo, a doctor in Montreal, a community leader in Nunavut, a factory worker in Halifax, a fashion designer in Toronto or a prairie farmer. More and more Canadians are embracing the midwifery option.

Every woman has her own reasons for choosing midwifery, but most of us still make our decisions about prenatal care and childbirth based on our own experience or that of our family and friends. If midwifery still seems inaccessible to many people, it may be because they don't know anyone who's tried it.

In our social circles, we were the first to choose the midwifery option.

For some of our friends and family, our decision seemed foreign and frightening. The questions started coming before our bellies began to bulge. As we grew, so did the list of queries. Over and over again, we discussed the safety of midwifery, our midwives' education, how they could deliver babies in homes or hospitals, how they were available to answer questions and urgent concerns at any time of the day or night.

Gradually, after hearing our replies and watching both moms and babies thrive in the excellent care of midwives, our families and friends came to understand our choices. Based on our wonderful experiences, many women we know have since opted for midwifery.

But the questions haven't stopped. Although we've each had two babies with the help of midwives, people are still asking. Neighbours, uncles-to-be, future grandmas, friends of friends of friends . . . They call. They come over. They stop us on the street. They want to know if midwifery is safe, if mothers have a high threshold for pain, and what happens in an emergency. They want to know how midwives will handle prenatal testing, how to keep their partners involved in their pregnancy, or how to support their friends in labour.

After we talk, most people feel reassured and more interested than ever in midwifery. Others still think we're brave or radical or naïve.

Of course, we're not any of these things. We're just informed. That's what it's all about. In Canada, it's a midwife's mandate to keep her client informed about her care and the choices available to her. Whether you're already working with a midwife or are just considering your options, this book will help you to be a full participant in your care. It will provide information, ideas and questions to discuss with your support people so that you can find answers of your own.

# How to Read this Book

As we will constantly assert in this book, midwifery care is about making informed choices and getting respect from your caregivers for the choices you make. As midwifery consumers, our choices were to attempt to give birth at home. As people, our choices were to have children in the context of long-term heterosexual partnerships. This will be apparent, as we can only write about our experiences from our particular perspectives.

Many women and men (midwives, mothers and fathers, grandmothers and grandfathers, even friends and extended family) were interviewed for this book. In doing so, we have tried to illustrate a wide range of experiences that women have had in midwifery care. We believe that it is important to reflect that midwifery care appeals to people from every part of our multi-faceted society, whether they be fundamentalist Christians, single parents, orthodox Jews, disabled, Native Canadians, immigrants, lesbians, teens, Muslims, surrogate parents. . . . It is impossible to name all the different types of women who choose midwifery. If you do not find a story from someone like yourself in this book, it does not mean that you won't find support in the care of midwives.

The stories are positioned in the book to highlight the themes in any given section. Sometimes the stories are broken into short anecdotes and the same storyteller may appear in the book several times. Sometimes a birth story appears in its entirety. This approach means that the stories may break up the flow of the book. If you'd like to go straight to the stories, or avoid them altogether, look for the grey bar that appears alongside each story or anecdote.

You may note that in most places in this book, we use the term *partner* to refer to both males and females. In order to protect their privacy, we use only the first names of the people who have generously shared their stories with us. Although we spoke to many midwives while doing the research for this book, we have not mentioned any of them by name. Our aim is not to provide advice from specific midwives but rather to give information about what your experience will be like if you choose midwifery care.

To give you some new and sometimes alternative information, at the end of each chapter we have provided references to several books that deal with midwifery, prenatal care and childbirth. However, their inclusion does not necessarily mean that we endorse them.

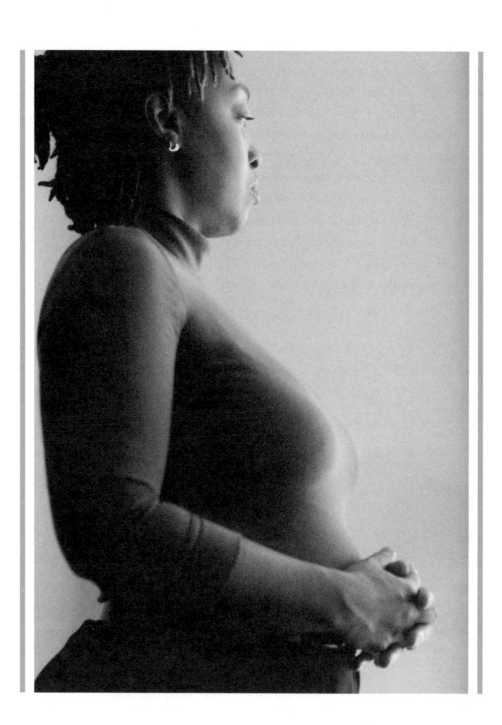

# One

## Choosing Midwifery

*Midwifery*. Whether it's because of the word itself or because of a lack of current or accurate information, many Canadians still see midwifery as either mysterious and foreign or quaint and unnecessary. To others, *midwife* is as ordinary a word as *nurse* or *doctor* or *grandmother*.

Midwifery, as it's practised in Canada, actually fits very well with our modern standard of individual choice. The practice of midwifery is equally at home in Mennonite communities and urban neighbourhoods, in the suburbs and in Inuit villages.

### What a Canadian Midwife Is

*What Midwife Means*

The term *midwife* is from the Old English meaning "with (mid) woman (wif)."

*What Midwives Do*

Midwives are primary care providers for women in all stages of pregnancy, birth and postpartum.

They are also responsible for newborn care in the first six weeks of life.

They work independently from the medical profession, but, in most places, midwives work within the established health care system, and they collaborate with physicians when necessary. Midwives usually work in a team with other midwives, though in some places they may employ a nurse or other appropriately trained person to act as an assistant (or second attendant) during birth.

Midwives are specialists in normal pregnancies and births, as defined by provincial midwifery legislation and the guidelines created by the provincial colleges that regulate midwifery.

In legislated areas midwives are able to prescribe and administer some drugs used during pregnancy and childbirth.

### How Midwives Are Educated

The first Canadian midwifery education programs were established in Ontario in 1993. Universities in three provinces now offer training in midwifery. These programs include intensive practical placements in which students practise under the supervision of midwives. Midwives who practise in provinces without educational programs generally receive their training in other ways. Some pursue a course of self-directed study and apprenticeship. Some come to midwifery with a background in maternal and obstetric nursing and then serve an apprenticeship. Others train and practise outside of Canada or in other provinces. In some provinces there are special provisions for aboriginal midwifery education that acknowledge the long-standing tradition of midwifery in the cultures of Canada's First Nations.

Midwives who come to Canada after training in other countries may be able to obtain their Canadian credentials by applying for registration. They may receive certification to practise in their home province. Depending on where they live, this may involve an assessment of their skills or a period of supervised practice. Once they have successfully completed this process, their skills meet provincial standards.

Like doctors, midwives who practise in provinces with midwifery legislation are governed by a professional college. The colleges set the standards for care and ensure that these standards are met. In provinces where midwifery is not legislated midwives are usually voluntarily governed through a professional association.

### Justine appreciates the hospital option

I went into labour at about 1:00 A.M. on Friday. We dozed on and off until 5:00 A.M., when it seemed futile to try to sleep any more. After letting the midwives know we were in labour, Patrick and I spent all of Saturday keeping a low profile at home, waiting for the contractions to speed up. It wasn't until about 10:30 P.M. that we phoned the midwives again to report contractions close enough together and intense enough for them to come over.

When the midwives arrived at our house, they determined that I was about four centimetres dilated, so we left for the hospital. I was a bit uncertain about whether to go, knowing it would be painful to ride in a car at that point, but in the end I felt glad we went. We were given a huge room with a Jacuzzi, and I was able to move around freely throughout the night without worrying about making a mess.

At the hospital, I used just about every birthing method available: the bed, the bed with the exercise ball, the birthing stool, the Jacuzzi, the toilet, walking with Patrick holding me up during contractions, lying on my back, and lying on the floor. By 7:00 A.M. my midwife thought it was time to call in the other midwife. This was a relief because the rest of us were exhausted, and she walked in refreshed.

From then on, it was a blur of pain and I felt an intense need for support and encouragement from Patrick and the team to endure and to continue to believe I could give birth my way. In the last hour and a half, I moved from the toilet to the Jacuzzi to the birthing stool, and finally onto all fours, which was the position the baby was born in. During this final stage, Patrick held me up to relieve the pressure on my tail bone, let me crush his fingers during contractions, and offered encouragement through each and every push, helping me to visualize my way through them.

What still amazes me is how well the baby did: his heartbeat remained strong as

I laboured to push him out. When he was born, he cried immediately; he squirmed and wriggled around just as he had done inside me for the past months. As soon as we were lying down, he latched on and was feeding just 20 minutes later. This activity helped me to deliver the placenta and served as a great distraction as I was stitched up (he was born with his hand beside his head, causing a small rip).

The other amazing thing was how alert and focused he seemed. A few hours after the birth, our families came to the hospital and then accompanied us home, and even with all the people around, he concentrated on us when we would start to speak.

I feel so gratified that we were able to do the birth our way.

—*Justine, mother of one*

## What a Midwife Isn't

### A Doctor

A doctor is trained to be the primary caregiver for all sorts of medical conditions. One of the areas in which he or she will be trained is pregnancy, birth and postpartum care. Some doctors will deliver babies as part of their general practice. Other doctors will specialize in prenatal care, birth and postpartum care, becoming obstetricians. These specialists are trained to handle complicated pregnancies and births.

### A Doctor's Assistant

Midwives in Canada do not function as doctors' assistants or as secondary care providers. The two professions work independently. Occasionally, women will have the care of a doctor as well as a midwife, either because they live in areas where midwives do not have access to lab tests and ultrasounds, or because of complications during pregnancy or birth that require consultation with a physician.

### A Nurse

A nurse receives training in all types of patient care and treatment. A part of that training will be in the area of labour, delivery and postpartum care. Some nurses will go on to specialize in obstetrics or pediatrics through on-the-job training.

In the United States, professionals called nurse-midwives deliver babies in birth centres or hospitals. A number of Canadian midwives have trained and worked as obstetric nurses but now practise midwifery exclusively. In some remote areas where physicians are not available, midwives (with or without nursing training) provide care.

### A Doula

A doula is a professional assistant who supports the mother during labour and acts as her advocate during birth. Some doulas will also aid the mother postpartum by helping to look after the baby and by doing household chores. Doulas may also provide prenatal information and classes.

Doulas do not have professional standing at hospitals, and they cannot attend births on their own. Their training may be informal or it may involve up to two years of classes and workshops. The mother hires the doula, and costs are not covered by government health care plans.

### A Non-Professional

Occasionally, a woman in a community who has attended for her friends' and neighbours' births may use the title "midwife" informally. Some women who have been attending births for years but choose not to practise within a system or as a member of a professional body, take clients for homebirth, but this is not the type of midwife we refer to in this book or the kind that is recognized by the health care system, professional bodies or most clients.

In European societies, before the existence of medicine and doctors, pregnancy and childbirth were handled by skilled and experienced local women. With the rise of science and the birth of the medical profession in the thirteenth century, people were persuaded to abandon traditional birthing practices in favour of new scientific approaches. Midwives were discredited by the new medical profession, which demeaned their work by labelling it witchcraft.

## Midwives and Choice

Midwives work hard to build a mother's confidence in her body's ability to give birth. They also respect women's choices. Canadian midwives are guided by a principle called "informed choice." Informed choice means you have the right to make decisions about your care, based on the information given to you by experienced professionals—in this case midwives. Thus the responsibility for the pregnancy is shared between the woman and her midwives.

In some ways, informed choice can be a daunting concept. If no one is going to make the decisions for you, you must be involved in your own care. Once you get used to the idea, though, it is very liberating. You can feel confident that what happens to you and your child will not be the result of coercion or a lack of information.

A perfect example that often arises is prenatal testing. Many tests are now standard in prenatal care. But standard does not mean mandatory. In one extreme case, Miranda encountered a pregnant woman who believed that it is illegal to refuse amniocentesis if you are over 35. Of course, this is not true. Prenatal testing is always an option for any pregnant woman, though it may not always be presented that way.

With midwives, you can rest assured that any choices are presented as such. The midwife's job is to provide the information, then let you select your option. Informed choice also means that midwives are there to support the choice you have made. Midwives do not offer interventions routinely. However, should the need for such assistance arise, the midwife will facilitate access to it.

Informed choice has its limits. If safety becomes an issue, midwives will give clear recommendations. In her first pregnancy, Sarah wanted to give birth at home. However, her medical condition was such that it seemed safer to deliver in the hospital. Her midwives told her that that was where they would need to attend to her and her baby. For Sarah, it was a very disappointing change in plans, but she understood that if there had been any options the midwives would have presented them. Even in the event of complications, midwives treat their clients with respect and explain every available choice. Thus the client knows that the restrictions are truly necessary and not just a convenience, a convention or a caregiver's own preference.

### Sarah's midwife–doctor health care team

In the first six months of my pregnancy, I felt great. Everything went the way I thought it would. I did have a little bleeding in my first trimester, but it turned out to be of no concern. My appointments with the midwife were filled with questions, stories and laughter. Then, in my twenty-seventh week, while on a weekend visit to Ottawa, I was immobilized by a painful swollen leg. I paged my midwife, who told me, very calmly, to go to the closest emergency department and explain that I might have a blood clot. I did and I spent the day waiting to be seen. Eventually, I had an ultrasound, but it didn't reveal any complications and I was allowed to leave.

When I called the midwife to tell her what had happened, she said that I should get a second opinion as soon as possible. The next day I went back to the hospital and had another ultrasound. This time the clot was obvious. I ended up having to stay at the hospital for a week.

I was in tremendous pain, and very frightened at times. But my midwife and the midwifery student stayed in close contact with me, asking me about the care I was receiving and making appointments for me to see specialists when I got home. They helped me understand what was happening and let me know what kinds of questions I should ask. The student, in particular, took time to find out more about my condition and gave me as much information as possible so that I could understand how the blood clot would affect my pregnancy and birth.

Once my condition became stable, I was able to return to Toronto, on crutches. There are not many sights sadder than a very pregnant woman on crutches in the winter! I met with my midwife right away and she explained how my care would proceed. First I would have to see a hematologist for the duration of the pregnancy and after the baby was born. As well, I would have to have a consultation about my care with an obstetrician specializing in high-risk cases. This obstetrician would confer with my midwife, the hematologist and me.

Once everyone had spoken to one another, we agreed that my care would be shared by both the midwives and the doctors for the rest of the pregnancy. In this model, I was mainly under the care of my midwives, but I also saw the doctors regularly. It might sound as if my condition meant that I lost the ability to make choices about my care. I did, in fact, have to give up my hope for a homebirth. But there were constant opportunities for my midwife and student to explain certain procedures and outcomes and to give me and my partner, Pete, occasions to be responsible for our care.

On one memorable day, at 32 weeks into my pregnancy, I had to rush to the hospital with Pete because I was bleeding. Our midwife met us there and explained that the doctor would do an examination to ascertain whether I was in early labour. If I was, then certain things would happen. She wanted to be sure that we knew what was coming. While she acknowledged that it was frightening, she made sure we had the support and information we needed in order to make the best possible decisions for both me and the baby. Because nothing that happened was unexpected, we were able to face the potential outcomes with courage.

Each time I faced a new problem or test, my midwife explained what our options were and what the test was for. Together we would try to figure out ways to help me have the natural and normal birth I wanted as well as a stress-free postpartum period. The midwives were advocates for me and my baby when I most needed them. Informed choice meant I could approach my birth and the numerous difficulties I faced with confidence.

—*Sarah, mother of two*

## Evidence-Based Practice

Many midwives in Canada use an "evidence-based practice" approach. This means the information they use to provide a woman and her family with choices is based on the latest research on a given topic, as well as on the client's preferences and values.

This approach means that midwives are lifelong learners who constantly take in an array of evidence. This involves assessing new research literature, learning on the job from peers and other professionals, asking clients direct and pertinent questions, and engaging in reflective practice that requires re-evaluating their own approaches to care. Midwives are taught to assess all of the evidence for its merit, applicability and effectiveness.

What this means for you is that your midwives will ask you questions in order to understand your physiological and personal needs. Since research constantly evolves, a midwife's advice might change from your first to your second pregnancy. What won't change is that you will be given a range of information on each topic drawn from research literature and your midwife's experience. In some cases, midwives may offer choices about care, based on pros and cons from the research. In other cases midwives may recommend a course of action or have practice protocols that guide the care they usually provide, based on the best available evidence. Ultimately, the decision lies with you and will reflect your own values and specific needs.

To be really effective, midwives need feedback about the care they provide. You can offer feedback during your visits or find other ways of giving your midwives and student midwives constructive criticism and other information about things that really worked for you. The midwives will use the information you and other families provide to do the following: develop practice protocols and regulations for best practice; conduct further research; approach hospitals about making positive changes; and advocate on behalf of childbearing women and families in the wider community.

## Is Midwifery Safe?

Midwives are specialists in normal birth. They bring both education and experience to the job.

Midwife-assisted births have comparable or lower rates of interventions than those births occurring in the medical system. This may be due in part to the fact that midwives attend lower-risk women. It is also because midwives work to avoid interventions, and so the incidence of complications from interventions is far lower.

During labour, midwives attend the women they have cared for prenatally. They know the specific details of your pregnancy as well as your wishes, and this helps them react to any situations that may arise during the birth.

Sometimes complications occur during pregnancy or birth that make medical advice or assistance necessary. Midwives get this assistance by conferring with a physician. The result may be that the woman's care is transferred entirely to an obstetrician. At other times, an obstetrician will offer recommendations for the woman's care, but the ultimate responsibility for putting these into effect lies with the midwives. Or, the midwife and obstetrician may work together for the duration of the pregnancy.

Women who experience complications in pregnancy or at birth particularly appreciate their midwifery care. The midwives play an active role in accessing resources and information, advocating on behalf of their client and explaining the nuances of her condition.

Both Sarah and Miranda had complications during their pregnancies that made consultations with a doctor necessary. But both continued as midwifery clients. During Sarah's first pregnancy, her care was shared by midwives and an obstetrician. But when she had her second baby, she simply consulted with physicians and was primarily cared for by her midwives.

## Midwifery and Pain

Every midwifery client has encountered people who assume that midwives are only for the brave. There is a misconception that midwifery clients feel more pain, since midwives believe that birth is a natural process requiring medical intervention only in the most difficult situations.

The majority of midwifery clients do not consider themselves brave or stoic. In fact, many people seek midwifery care precisely because they fear pain.

Study after study has shown that women in labour experience less pain when they are accompanied by a familiar attendant with training and experience. It lessens their fear. When fear diminishes, their experience of pain is substantially reduced.

Our midwives gave the following example: pain often occurs as a result of something that is wrong within the body—such as a broken arm or a burst appendix. The pain is heightened by our bodies and minds telling us it should not exist.

Fear intensifies the experience of pain.

The pain of labour is different. While it *is* intense, it is a working pain, which should exist. When you have attendants who see this pain as a productive means to an end, they can help you get through it without fear.

As you experience the challenges of labour, your midwives will continue to keep you informed, letting you know what is going on in your body and helping you recognize when there are choices to be made. Information and understanding are very helpful tools for managing pain.

When midwives attend your birth, you not only have familiar, trusted individuals at your side, you have familiar, trusted individuals with knowledge and experience. People who believe in your ability to have your baby your way. People who believe in your strength and competence. The midwives convey this confidence during birth, prenatally and when you become the mother of a newborn. They believe you can do it, and somehow, so do you.

Midwives are also adept at helping you manage pain in non-medical ways. They know how to use water, movement, sound and so on, to help you work your way through difficult times in labour. After nine months, they also know *you* well enough to understand what may get you through the hard parts.

However, midwives also have enough experience with labouring mothers to recognize that there is a point when interventions like pain relief are necessary and beneficial. For example, in a long labour, an epidural can help you get some needed rest and assist the process. In some cases it may help you avoid the much more serious outcome of a caesarean section. In other situations you may find that midwives will also encourage you to use pain relief and other interventions.

Though midwifery clients do not feel more pain than their peers who opt for a doctor-attended hospital birth, they also do not expect a pain-free experience. Most women, even those who use all sorts of drugs, do feel at least some pain during labour and delivery. Midwives do not try to hide the fact that labour is painful and challenging. But they promise to help you through it every step of the way.

### Laurie faces her fear of pain

Like all women who wait until relatively late in life to have children, I had many reasons to delay. But if I am really honest with myself, I have to admit that one of the main reasons I waited till age 35 was fear of childbirth. I don't think my fear was run-of-the-mill. I was absolutely terrified of the pain and I felt overwhelmed by my fear.

Fortunately, my friend Elizabeth told me about midwifery. She believed that if I could stop being so frightened, the pain would be bearable. She said no doctor, no matter how kind, would have the time to talk me through my fears. "But what about pain relief?" I wanted to know. My friend said, "You'll see. Midwives have a big bag of tricks."

So I made an appointment to talk to a midwife. When she asked me why I was interested in midwifery, I was blunt. I didn't care what music played in the background or what the birthing room looked like. I was not interested in midwifery because I was determined to have a natural, drug-free birth. I just wanted to survive the experience without biting off my tongue!

My midwife explained that epidurals may actually slow down a naturally progressing labour and can lead to complications in birth, so I started to listen more closely. Women labouring in a safe, nurturing environment, under the guidance of people they know and trust, tend to be able to manage pain more easily, my midwife explained. There are also breathing techniques and labouring positions that can ease the pain, she added.

But what if something went wrong and I was going out of my mind with pain? Would relief be denied? I wondered. The answer was the clincher for me: "If you do need more help from drugs and technology, if you or your baby need medical assistance, you will get it."

My midwife told me that when I went into labour she and another midwife would come to the house to help us decide when to go to the hospital. They wear pagers and are available day or night. There seemed to be no downside. Maybe I could actually do this, I thought.

My son was born in the hospital after 12 hours of labour. The pain was there, but proved manageable without drugs. With my husband and midwives at my side, I wasn't gripped by the terror of the unknown that I had feared for so many years. My second child blasted her way into the world in less than two hours. Her birth was much more intense and painful. But I never lost my mind or bit my tongue off!

Looking back on two natural childbirths assisted by midwives, I can't imagine how anyone has a baby without this type of care. In addition to having had two spectacular birthing experiences, I am surprised to say that I have also gained a new trust in my body. The mystery of childbirth no longer terrifies me. It leaves me in awe of the female body.

—*Laurie, mother of two*

## The Midwifery Difference

Throughout this book and in any conversation you may have with midwives, you will notice that a distinctly different terminology is used to refer to the mother and birth. Doctors have patients. Midwives have clients. Doctors deliver babies. Midwives "catch" them.

The midwives' approach to care is to leave the power in the woman's hands and to acknowledge that she is the one doing the work and experiencing the joy and pain of labour, childbirth and parenthood. From the terminology on, midwives attempt to build a relationship with the women in their care and the women's own networks of support (partner, family and friends).

### Talking and listening at midwives' appointments

Everything about the care I received during my second pregnancy was so civilized! Tests were explained in full, and we were given options, backed up with statistics and studies. We would sit around on the couch and talk about dreams, fears, food, and sexuality, whatever our concerns were. I felt no trepidation phoning with a question and was given books and videotapes on loan if I was interested. My entire being was the focus, not just the pregnancy. Near the end of my pregnancy, we spent several hours talking about different methods and techniques my partner and I could use to relieve pain. Mostly my midwives made me feel strong and able to do this confidently.

—*Carolyn, mother of two*

This starts with the time they take to listen to questions, concerns and stories. Midwives' visits tend to last longer than doctor's appointments (45 minutes is the average), which allows you to get to know each other, and gives the midwife plenty of time to familiarize herself with the particulars of your pregnancy.

### Informed and thoughtful care

The two doctors that we visited throughout our first pregnancy were very competent and friendly, but the typical 30-minute wait for a 5-minute appointment did not make us feel comfortable or confident. We read the books and talked to other people. We took the prenatal classes. Still, the total amount of time we spent with the woman who was eventually going to deliver our baby was not more than two hours.

Working with a midwife (or midwives, in our case) proved to be more human. It wasn't just hand holding, it was informed, thoughtful, human interaction.

—*Chris, father of two*

Midwives give their clients regular appointments, just as a family doctor or an obstetrician does. The standard pattern of appointments is usually one per month in the first and second trimester, and every two weeks in the third trimester until week 36. In the final month of your pregnancy, a midwife would see you weekly. In some regions the pattern of appointments may change slightly to accommodate more postnatal appointments or visits with second midwives.

Midwives in legislated areas offer their clients access to all the standard tests, just as a doctor would. They also explain the purpose and potential outcome of each test before you decide whether to take it.

While many obstetricians won't see you until the end of your first trimester, midwife visits begin as soon as you learn you are pregnant. That means that midwives are there to deal with morning sickness, nutrition and miscarriage. The longer visits, combined with the midwives' commitment to relationship building, leave you free to discuss your emotions about your pregnancy as well as its physical progression. This is a real advantage when it comes to dealing with your feelings about pregnancy loss, postpartum blues or conflicting feelings about impending parenthood.

Some midwives practise in offices, others practise out of their homes, and a few do visits only in the clients' homes. No matter where they are based, midwives are likely to visit your home on at least one occasion before you give birth. This gives them the opportunity to make sure they know how to get there when you go into labour, since most midwives will help their clients labour at home, even if the birth itself is planned for the hospital or birth centre. It also helps the midwives see you in your element and makes it easier for them to meet your support people.

### A comfortable atmosphere

I enjoyed the comfortable atmosphere of my midwife's office, which was in her home. It was decorated like a home, not a hospital room. What meant the most was the time she gave me to share my concerns, ask questions and just talk. I knew she cared about me, and I knew that she'd keep all my wishes in mind when it came to the birth.

—*Melanie, mother of two*

During the birth, midwives work in teams to offer the mother and child the best and safest care possible. When you give birth, two midwives (or in some cases a midwife with a trained assistant such as a nurse) will attend you. Your care will be the principal responsibility of one midwife; the other midwife will be primarily devoted to your baby. You will probably get to know both midwives at your appointments. You may also have the opportunity to meet other midwives as well as student midwives.

Unlike the majority of obstetricians (who deliver their patients' babies only if they are the doctor on call that shift), most midwifery practices guarantee someone you know will be at your birth. All practices have devised a system to cover weekends and midwives' holidays. At the Toronto practice that Miranda and Sarah have used, midwives take one weekend off per month and two full months off per year. At any practice, when your midwife is away, you will almost always be attended by another midwife you know.

In addition to offering longer appointments and being present at your birth, many midwives are available by pager, 24 hours a day. Most questions and worries can wait until office hours, but if you suspect you are in labour or have an urgent concern you should call. Your midwives will discuss paging protocols with you.

A few months into Miranda's first pregnancy, when she had to make frequent use of the pager service, her husband began to grasp the value of the care they were getting. When asked to describe midwifery, he called it "the most honourable profession."

### A nurturing relationship

I hired my midwife to provide a service: to support me through the possibility of another miscarriage, and, at best, to get me through a birth. I never anticipated the nurturing relationship that came with it.

—*Diane, mother of one*

Midwives are the consummate experts when it comes to support in labour. Most midwives can offer their clients a choice of birth at home or in hospital. No matter what place you choose to give birth, midwifery care usually means you get to spend much more time at home than in a hospital bed. Midwifery clients tend to go to the hospital later in labour than their counterparts who are under a doctor's care, and they are discharged a lot faster too—often within a few hours of giving birth.

That's because midwives make frequent home visits during the first two weeks of your child's life. They come to your house to help to establish breastfeeding and to ensure that your baby is thriving and you feel physically and mentally well. Again, they are usually available by pager to answer questions or respond to urgent concerns. If you require supplementary support such as pediatricians, lactation consultants or counsellors, midwives will take the time to find the right person for your needs. Many mothers say it is during these first few days at home with a newborn that they really see what midwifery has meant to their family.

# Midwifery: Frequently Asked Questions

*Who Do Midwives Attend?*

Midwifery is not a fringe phenomenon, nor does it appeal only to the educated middle class. Teenagers, older mothers, single parents, and members of religious, racial or cultural minorities seek midwifery care. Across class, race, culture and sexual orientation, every woman has her own reasons for choosing midwifery. But all midwifery clients are alike in the belief that midwifery will be better tailored to their own beliefs and desires than standard medical care.

### Breaking misconceptions

For me, it was important to see all the other women at my midwives' prenatal classes. I had this stereotype about the type of women choosing midwives—I thought that everyone would be less conservative than me. But there were so many different types of people! I learned so much, breaking that misconception.

—*Jessica, mother of two*

### A Canadian midwifery experience

I had my first two babies in Pakistan, in a hospital with a doctor in attendance.

When I got pregnant here in Canada I heard about midwives through a friend. I am Muslim and I wear a hijab, so it is forbidden for me to be seen by any male staff or doctors. This was a problem because even if I had a female doctor there was no guarantee that I would have a female doctor when I went into the hospital to deliver my baby.

I called the community health centre and they put me in contact with the midwives. I went to meet with them; they are so humble, so nice. I knew it was going to be good. I am going to have my baby in the hospital and they have told me that they will protect me from being seen by male staff. I am very satisfied with them and comfortable with them.

—*Zoofishan, mother of two*

It's true that there are some women with pre-existing medical conditions for whom midwifery would not be an option—the truly "high risk." But many women who assume they are in such a category are actually perfect candidates for midwifery. Being as young as 17 or as old as 40 does not automatically bar you from midwifery care. Neither does a history of miscarriages, a previous caesarean birth, problems with previous pregnancies or most physical disabilities. Midwifery care is about working with individual mothers. Only by assessing your unique set of concerns with a midwife can you determine whether you will be able to pursue care outside the medical profession.

### Disability and choice

I have a slight case of cerebral palsy, which causes me to limp and my pelvis to be slightly tilted. Having this disability worried me, since I wasn't sure how it would affect me when giving birth, and I really wanted to have a midwife. My friends and family were worried about the safety of my choice. But I have never let my disability stop me from trying to do things I think I am perfectly capable of doing, even if others are doubtful.

In the end I did choose midwifery care. The midwives reassured me that my disability had no bearing on childbirth, and that I was fully capable of giving birth naturally. I am very glad that I made this informed and educated choice. It was a beautiful experience; the midwives instilled me with confidence through their wonderful care.

—Brandie, mother of one

### Learning about today's midwifery

When I first learned I was pregnant I was in a state of shock. I felt surprised that this secret longing was actually being fulfilled and amazed that it could happen so easily. I was also terrified of this unknown path I had now set out upon. I had known about midwives from my youth in Winnipeg when I had befriended a community of young mothers (mostly single). They introduced me to the midwifery practice and home-birthing, which was quite strong in Winnipeg at that time, although it was still considered very "alternative." To me, it seemed the normal way of having babies.

Ten years later, I was living in Toronto. Having fallen out of touch with that community, I had no knowledge of the state of midwifery care in Ontario. I came across no obvious public information about it. I had no idea that it was funded by the government. I found out about midwifery because, as a pregnant woman, I had a vested interest in doing so. Then I had to start educating my family and friends about this generally little-known style of practice. Even my brother, an anesthesiologist, knew very little about it and felt suspicious of such an "archaic" practice.

In my ignorance, I also chose to seek medical care because spina bifida runs in my family and so there was a chance my baby might be born with it. I figured that this risk would require me to take a highly medical route anyway, so I might as well stick with my doctor at the hospital. But after seeing a genetic counsellor and having a normal 12-week ultrasound, I reconsidered and sought more information on midwives. The nurse practitioners at my hospital were very helpful with information and helping me make the transfer. It was afterwards that I learned I could have received the same referrals to a genetic counsellor through my midwife. I had no idea that they could share care in a risk pregnancy.

*—Erica, mother of one*

*Where Do Midwives Work?*

As of 2002, midwifery is legislated in the following provinces and territories: Alberta, British Columbia, Manitoba, Ontario, Quebec and Saskatchewan.

Midwives also provide care in some remote communities such as Rankin Inlet, Nunavut, and St. Anthony's, Newfoundland. In areas such as Nova Scotia and Yukon, there are active midwifery practices, but no official legislation for the profession. Though midwifery is not illegal in these areas, it is not yet an accepted or integrated part of the health care system.

*Where Do Midwives Attend Births?*

In most provinces with legislation, midwives offer their clients a choice of birth place. Usually this means choosing between home or hospital. In Quebec, midwifery clients give birth in freestanding birth centres.

*How Much Does Midwifery Cost?*

The cost of having a midwife-attended birth depends entirely on where you live. As of 2002, the entire bill is paid by the government in the following places: British Columbia; Manitoba; Rankin Inlet, Nunavut; Ontario and Quebec.

In other places, midwives are hired directly by the client, who is responsible for the bill. The cost of midwives' services ranges from pay-what-you-can to set fees, and varies from place to place. There are also some government-funded midwifery projects, such as a birthing centre in Rankin Inlet and northern Newfoundland. The success of these projects should lead to public funding of midwifery in more areas of the country.

**Affordable care**

I was cleaning houses, trying to make money, when I got pregnant. One of my clients knew I wasn't a landed immigrant yet and that I couldn't get health care, so she suggested I contact the midwives. I met them when I was three months along and they were able to help me. I could pay them what I could afford, a little at a time. I had that baby at home with their help. I had already had three babies at home in Jamaica with the help of a nurse-midwife, so it wasn't strange for me, or my family, to have the baby at home.

The midwives were so good. I called them when the water broke, and they were there with me the whole time. One of them massaged my back to make the pain go away. I have had the rest of my babies with the same midwives, and each birth has been different. The midwives were even with me when I had to have a C-section.

—*Beverley, mother of six*

*How Do You Find a Midwife?*

You can find a midwife by calling either the college of midwifery in your province, the midwifery association in your province, or local advocacy groups. These organizations are listed in the Appendix at the end of this book. You can find out more about midwifery and how it works across Canada in Chapter 2.

*Is It For You?*

What are you really signing up for when you choose midwifery? The following list summarizes the commitments most clients make when they choose midwifery care. They agree to:

- Become informed
- Participate in making decisions
- Attempt to give birth without routine use of pain relief or medical intervention
- Plan to breastfeed

Even if this sounds like something you would be interested in doing, you don't have to decide immediately. In keeping with their emphasis on information and choice, most midwives use the initial appointment with a client to talk about what midwifery means to the midwife and to the mother and her partner. Only by meeting your potential midwife, and discussing your particular wishes and needs, will you know if midwifery care is for you. Every woman's needs are different, and midwives adapt their approach to the individual's requirements and preferences.

I chose midwives because I wanted to be a participant rather than a patient.

—*Penny, mother of one*

On Miranda's first visit to her midwife, she appreciated the candour with which her midwife described the work ahead: "For many women, birth is simultaneously the best and the most challenging time in a woman's life."

Two babies and one miscarriage later, Miranda understands what most midwifery clients learn through their own experience: Midwives are there to hold your hand through both of these extremes and everything in between.

## ◈ *If You Want to Read More . . .*

*The Mother of All Pregnancy Books: An All-Canadian Guide to Conception, Birth & Everything in Between*, by Ann Douglas (Toronto: CDG Books, 2000).

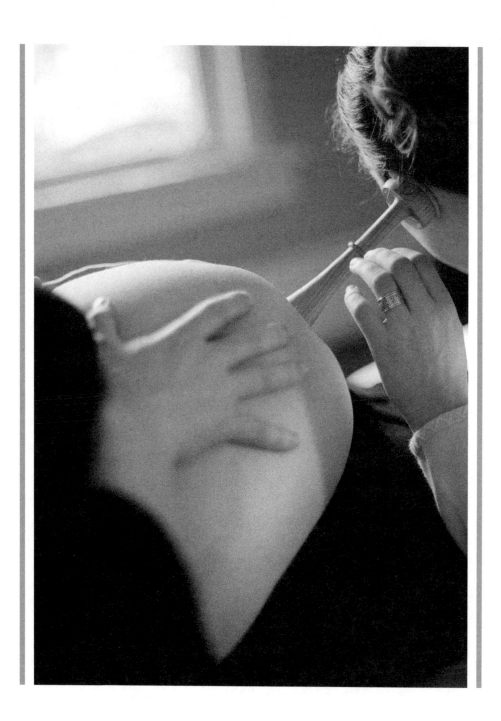

## Two

### Canadian Midwifery: Two Histories

If you watch Canadian television, you're probably familiar with Heritage Minutes—little vignettes that celebrate Canadian notables such as Nelly McClung and the guy who invented Superman. A few years ago, the Canadian midwife received her minute of fame. She doesn't leap tall buildings in a single bound, but she does manage to get to a labouring mother in the middle of a Canadian winter, despite the dark and a sled stuck in the snow.

It's nice to see a little bit of good publicity for the Canadian midwife, who still battles the myths and misconceptions established in the days shortly after that fictitious midwife abandoned her sled to reach a woman who needed her.

But to consider the history of Canadian midwifery it is necessary to distinguish the tradition of birth attendants among the immigrant settlers from the almost uninterrupted history of midwifery among Canada's First Nations.

### Inuit and First Nations Midwifery

Every culture has its own way of providing support and expertise to women when they give birth. Among the communities that populated Canada before the arrival of white settlers, knowing how to aid mothers during birth was probably a skill shared by both women and men. The nomadic life of these communities meant that the population was sometimes fragmented. If birth attendance was a shared skill, then expectant mothers were assured an experienced, knowledgeable assistant when they went into labour, regardless of the season or the circumstances.

### Refusing to leave home

I chose to stay here. When we were young, we used to play "giving birth" with our dolls. I knew that someday I was going to have a baby without leaving my town. All the women used to leave for Montreal and Moose Factory. When I started to see the prenatal workers, I told them I was going to stay here no matter what they said, and I kept my word. The maternity centre in Puvirnituq was already open. I knew if women started staying in Inukjuak, a maternity centre would open faster here.

In the last two months of my pregnancy, they sent me to Puvirnituq for an X-ray to check if the baby's head was down. They asked the midwives there to try to convince me to stay. But the midwives didn't even try because I told them point-blank I wouldn't go anywhere no matter how much they tried. I had to accomplish my dream of staying in my community to have my baby. My son was born here, in Inukjuak. There were no midwives, just prenatal and postnatal workers.

—*Brenda, mother of one*

In the late 1800s and early 1900s in the settled south of Canada, the federal government assisted in the disintegration of midwifery by agreeing to make the practice illegal. Later, in the North, it took the opposite approach. First Nations people had been attending one another during labour for centuries. However, in an effort to provide medical services to the North, in the 1960s the federal government hired foreign-trained white midwives to provide birth services to aboriginal communities. First Nations women were brought into nursing stations to deliver their babies, while white women living in the area were flown to faraway hospitals days or weeks before their due dates. By the mid-1970s, in a push to provide equal services, aboriginal women were also being flown to distant hospitals. They went without their families and often against their will. As in other societies, the traditions of hundreds of years quickly crumbled.

Although midwifery was still being practised until relatively recently in First Nations communities, the women who provided this care were dying out. However, recent initiatives within some communities have shepherded in a new era of midwifery. In places such as Puvirnituq in northern Quebec and Six Nations in Ontario, birth centres staffed by aboriginal midwives blend long-standing traditions and practices with today's clinical knowledge.

### Birth among friends

I have four children and all of them were born in the North. Three of them were born in a small hospital in Puvirnituq, where my mother works as one of the midwives. My fourth baby was born in the maternity centre in Inukjuak. This meant I didn't have to get on a plane at the end of my pregnancy, I could walk around my home at the beginning of labour.

I was scared to have the babies, but once I was in the maternity centre, I felt safe. I would not want to have to go to the south to have a baby, because it would take me away from my family and I would be homesick. Having a baby at home, in the community with family around, is so special.

*—Syra, mother of four*

## Midwifery Around the World

*Who Is Catching Babies around the World?*

People often react with surprise when they hear that women in many parts of the world have never even thought of having a doctor attend their births. But midwives are considered experts in childbirth the world over. One estimate is that 75 percent of the world's children are born into the hands of midwives. In England, 70 percent of babies are caught by midwives. In Holland, one-third of all babies are born at home with the aid of midwives, and 90 percent of babies are born with midwives in attendance. In fact, until the early 1990s, Canada was one of only a handful of countries that had no midwifery legislation.

In some parts of the world, midwives' expertise in birth has never been challenged, and midwifery has always been accepted as the profession that grew out of women's need to be attended during labour. But in others, mainly in Europe and subsequently in North America, midwives have had to struggle to attain their current professional standing. In some countries, two factors—the rise of the physician and the fourteenth-century witch hunts in Europe—caused a breakdown in the reputation and practice of midwifery, which is only now being fully repaired.

When medical education became formalized in Europe in the thirteenth century, doctors were compelled to train in a university. But because access was limited to men, any women practicing medicine were labelled ignorant because of their lack of formal education, or were perceived as misrepresenting themselves in their qualifications. The first people to employ the newly trained doctors for birth were royalty. For everyone else, a midwife was the person you turned to in childbirth or illness. The women who attended mothers in labour were also skilled herbalists who provided remedies for a variety of ailments.

The new class of educated and professional healing men realized that, in order to gain the confidence of the people, they would have to discredit

> **Saying *midwife* around the world**
>
> Czech – *porodni baba* – "birthing grandmother"
>
> Danish – *jorde moder* – "earth mother"
>
> Dutch – *vroedvrouw* – "wise woman"
>
> French – *sage-femme* – "wise woman"
>
> German – *Hebamme* – "old woman who picks up newborns"
>
> Hebrew – *m'yaledet* – "one who helps with birth"
>
> Hindi – *daii* – "one who places the baby"
>
> Inuktitut – *Ikajuqti* – "assistant at birth"
>
> Japanese – *san ba* – "old woman at birth"
>
> Mandarin – *jie shen p'o* – "older woman who helps other woman to have a baby"
>
> Nishnawbe, Ojibway – *do-di-seem* – "one who cuts the cord"
>
> Portuguese – *parteira* – "birther"
>
> Russian – *a kyme pka* – "mother cutting the umbilical cord"
>
> Sanskrit – *saavikaa* – "one who assists in birth"
>
> Swahili – *m-kunga* – "confidential advisor, especially an older friend who gives advice"
>
> Vietnamese – *co do de* – "woman who supports birth"

the work of traditional healers. The Middle Ages were also marked by the Church's attempts to root out the pagan traditions that stood in the way of the Church's supremacy. And so midwives and women healers became the target of witch hunts, in which thousands of women were burned or drowned in the name of religion.

Women still needed birth attendants, however, so midwifery continued. Most people could not afford to hire a doctor, and childbirth was considered a women's "ailment" that was of little interest to most medical men. Attending births was time-consuming and not very profitable. Moreover, their medical education gave them little training in the birth process. But doctors' role in birth began to change around 1600 when an English barber-turned-obstetrician by the name of Peter Chamberlen invented a tool designed to pull the baby out of the birth canal. This tool was called forceps. Many doctors wanted to employ the new technology, but its use was limited to the Chamberlen family. The family kept the design a secret for another 100 years, becoming wealthy in the process. Eventually, the use of forceps and similar innovations became widespread. However, the law allowed only doctors to use them. As doctors embraced a more active role in labour management, they began adding births to their list of services, and midwives came to be viewed as outdated, and as having limited abilities.

## Midwifery in Early Canada

In the seventeeth century, thousands of European immigrants were lured to the future Canada by the promise of a better life. But many of them ended up facing hardship. The land they settled was often far away from any established community, and the nearest neighbours might also be hours away in good weather. This meant that a labouring mother faced giving birth without the assistance of family and friends from home, and perhaps without any assistance whatsoever.

Certainly, among the immigrants there would be women who had become skilled birth attendants in their countries of origin, but what were the chances of such women living next door? The women who helped the new Canadians give birth were probably mothers or grandmothers, experienced in aiding their own small circle. It is most likely that they didn't call themselves midwives or assume midwifery as a profession. Research suggests that most women voluntarily assisted their pregnant neighbours, knowing that the favour would be returned when they themselves needed help—whether in birth or harvesting crops or raising a barn.

Even if they didn't claim midwifery as a profession, these birth attendants must have had ample opportunity to catch babies. Large families were the norm, and would probably have included the birth attendant's own brood of at least six children.

The technical assistance that these midwives could provide the birthing women was limited. Any "surgical" procedure they undertook would be in order to save a mother's life when there was no longer any hope for a happy outcome for both mother and baby. But accounts from the time indicate a few tried-and-true non-surgical techniques used to get the baby out. Some women were adept at massaging the uterus to turn babies who were in a breech position, making for an easier delivery. The use of different birth positions, such as a squat, was also common to encourage the baby along. "Quilling" involved filling a quill with cayenne pepper and blowing it up the mother's nose. The violent sneezing would help her push the baby out.

Like today's midwives, the birth attendant was an important support in the postpartum period. After the baby was born, the birth attendant and other neighbours and friends would help to make sure the rest of the family was fed and that the mother had a few days' bedrest before she was thrown back into the strenuous day-to-day routine of hauling water, cooking, baking, ironing, sewing and taking care of children.

## The Doctor Migration

Drawn by the growing communities, immigrants with professional qualifications also arrived in Canada. Among the arrivals were newly trained doctors. Areas that experienced early development and prosperity were introduced to doctors before the more far-flung settlements. Though European-trained doctors first began arriving in the early 1700s, in many communities doctors were a rarity until well into the twentieth century.

Doctors brought many needed skills to Canada, but birth expertise doesn't seem to have been one of them. Many doctors arrived having attended only four births—the number that was required in order to graduate from European medical schools. Still, the doctors came with bags containing forceps and chloroform, and the intention to make birth a profitable part of their practice.

In the name of progress, some women accepted the doctor's new role in birth, but many resisted, for a variety of reasons. Doctors usually had to travel farther than the neighbouring farm, and would often miss the birth altogether. Women birthing in Canada were used to being attended by women, but doctors were all men. Midwives had techniques born out of experience. The midwives of the day understood the women's poverty and the demands made on them in the home, because they shared these domestic responsibilities. The midwives were the mothers' friends. The doctors were "professionals" at a time when this meant a social division as well as an economic one. And attendance at birth, once provided at no cost or at a minimal charge, was now a billable service.

Some doctors invested in their communities by assisting at births alongside the local women who were birth attendants. These doctors' willingness to learn and the respect they showed for their patients increased the likelihood that they would eventually be embraced by their communities. But not everyone was ready to accept the doctor as a new and necessary part of birthing. The reluctance to move away from women-attended births began to be referred to as "the midwife problem." The doctors successfully petitioned the governments of the day to make midwifery illegal. In Ontario in 1865, midwifery came under the jurisdiction of licensed medical practitioners. This meant that any woman attending at a birth could be charged with "practising medicine without a licence." Midwives were rarely charged, but the threat of arrest and prosecution deterred many women from providing midwifery services.

In addition, public health campaigns promoted the image of local birth attendants as uneducated and unfit for the job. Midwives were dirty. Midwives had no experience. Midwives meant pain. Midwives were drunks. Midwives had no training in the use of the latest technologies.

From early on, this message was spread by doctors in the areas where they practised. It later became part of an educational effort on a more national scale. From about 1920, nurses who had completed their training in hospitals went to small communities across the West to provide public health education. One of their primary tasks was to remind people that midwives were not appropriate birth attendants and that it was illegal for them to practise. Radio broadcasts instructed women to submit completely to their doctor in matters regarding birth.

Two technological inventions also helped doctors assume responsibility for the birth process: the car and the hospital. The car made it possible for doctors to attend more patients in a day and to reach patients who were previously out of their jurisdiction. As patients themselves began to buy automobiles, even many rural patients were able to come to the city-based doctor, and the era of birth in hospital began.

Voices and information that contradicted the medical profession's line were not heard publicly. In 1940, a manual published by the federal government called *The Canadian Mother and Child* included helpful information on birth without a doctor for women in unserviced areas. The author, Dr. Ernest Couture, was later chastised by the medical community, and subsequent editions ensured that this message got out: birth without a doctor in attendance was unsafe and illegal. By the late 1940s, despite the fact that midwives were still practising in Canada, especially in isolated areas, all references to midwifery in this manual had disappeared.

Also suppressed were studies conducted in the 1920s and 1930s that showed doctor-led births and births in hospitals had poorer results than births at home, with or without doctors. In 1919, the Medical Officer of Health for Saskatchewan had reported that pregnant women in Saskatchewan who were not attended by a physician in birth were at a greatly reduced risk of dying in childbirth. In the hopes of making a case for hospitals in isolated areas, the Red Cross conducted a survey in 1928. But it revealed that more mothers died giving birth in hospital than at home. The biggest risk factor in hospital was the likelihood of epidemics and outbreaks of bacterial infections. Neither of these studies was made available to the public or even to most doctors. The medical profession continued to tell mothers, fathers and its own members that women who chose to avoid doctors at birth were putting both their own health and their babies' health at risk.

Some doctors continued to attend births at home, despite the message that hospital births were safer. For some, this was due to their own beliefs and experience showing positive outcomes for homebirth. For others, hospital birth was impossible or impractical due to a lack of local facilities. Mona, Sarah's partner's mother, was born at home in southern Ontario, as were her seven siblings between 1924 and 1940. Mona remembers her dad getting the cutter out on more than one occasion in the depth of winter so that he could fetch the doctor. Mona's mother also received assistance during labour and through the postpartum period from a local woman. Mona's mother would typically stay in bed for a few days after giving birth, and Mona remembers being allowed in to the bedroom to inspect the new baby and seeing how happy her mother looked. The ninth, and last, child was born in hospital.

The acceptance of midwife-attended births was eroded in a little more than a generation. Although midwifery and homebirth, especially in isolated, First Nations or religious communities were still practised, midwives themselves became increasingly socially isolated. In later years, however, the absence of a doctor often had less to do with choice and more to do with the mother's financial situation. Though midwives were maligned and ridiculed, though they were barred from birth by the threat of legal action, most doctors would only assist at homes where the family could afford their fee. As the midwives were driven out, many women went unattended during labour because they couldn't afford to pay. Birth without anyone in attendance was not an illegal act.

Birthing without a doctor, and eventually birthing at home, came with a stigma of poverty and ignorance. Even those born safely at home, like Mona, came to believe that homebirth was an inferior and dangerous choice.

## The Rebirth of Midwifery

If the image of the dirty, uneducated midwife does not still linger in many Canadians' minds, it is likely because it has been supplanted by the image of the long-haired hippie. And modern midwifery does owe a great deal to the hippie—or "natural living," or "back to the land"—movements of the 1960s and 1970s. These social movements challenged institutions and technology and raised questions in the minds of many expectant parents. And once again a media push, this time with a pro-midwife slant, caught the attention of some mothers and fathers.

The media in question were mostly books from Europe and North America, which revealed the grisly nature of hospital births at the time—stirrups, forceps, unnecessary C-sections, complications from the overuse of drugs, shaving, enemas, episiotomies, forced separation of mother and infant. The new literature, by authors such as Ina May Gaskin, Sheila Kitzinger and Frederick Leboyer, reminded readers that there was another way, a way that had been working very well until about the last one hundred years.

Birthing mothers who wanted to avoid the medicalized experience at the hospital started seeking alternatives. The most obvious option was to plan to have their children at home. Some were confident enough to enlist only their partner's help during labour and birth, but most wanted the additional assistance of birth attendants. In some communities, a doctor or nurse or midwife trained in another country was willing to attend births outside the hospital, but such professionals were difficult to find, and they always faced the danger of being ostracized by other members of their professions.

Many women who were determined to avoid intervention settled for support but not experience, calling on friends and neighbours who expressed an interest in the idea of birth without technology or interference. To prepare, some of these invited attendants studied obstetrical texts, but others came equipped only with their ideals. Many were inspired by their attendance at the births of family and friends, and they saw a need for birth attendants who were experienced and knowledgeable and yet believed in the natural process of birth. In short, they recognized their future vocations.

Gradually these women acquired a knowledge of the birth process by reading textbooks and by observing. They found one another and shared their knowledge. They began to expand their services beyond their own circles to care for other like-minded mothers who had heard about their approach. There is insufficient documentation to assess how many women practised in this way or to provide statistics for the number of babies who were born with their assistance. What we do know is that these women became the first of Canada's new midwives.

> **Books that inspired a movement**
>
> *Childbirth Without Fear* by Grantly Dick-Read
>
> *Birth Without Violence* by Frederick Leboyer
>
> *Spiritual Midwifery* by Ina May Gaskin
>
> *Birth Reborn* by Michael Odent
>
> *The Experience of Childbirth* by Sheila Kitzinger
>
> *The Birth Book* by Raven Lang
>
> *Immaculate Deception* by Suzanne Arms

## Transition to a New Midwifery

Despite the satisfaction of parents attended by these new midwives, this profession proved difficult on many levels. The pay was poor. Midwives sometimes worked for free and often accepted barter or minimal payment for prenatal, birth and postpartum care. It was difficult to attain an education: to become a well-trained practitioner, aspiring midwives had to find experienced and willing midwives with whom to pursue a self-directed apprenticeship. And there was the ever-present threat of being charged with practising medicine without a licence.

Though the families that hired midwives had made a commitment to avoid unnecessary interventions at birth, the fact that midwives lacked access to the medical system was an ongoing challenge. Should a woman in labour require medical assistance, the midwives had no privileges at the hospital. A woman's midwife might be allowed into the hospital to act as a support person, but it was just as likely she would be denied entry by hospital staff. In some areas midwives had sympathetic doctors they could call on to help their clients; but for the most part midwives could expect that they, and their clients, would be treated with suspicion. It was highly unlikely that anyone would take a pregnant woman's history from the midwife who accompanied her, and there were instances of labouring women being refused necessary medical care because they had hired a midwife.

Midwives also found that some women who wanted the midwifery option were not willing or able to opt for birth at home. For women with certain medical conditions or histories, quick access to medical care was necessary, and a homebirth was not a wise option. Increasingly, midwives debated how best to serve these clients without compromising their care. Sometimes they acted as labour support in hospital, and at other times they reluctantly turned women away. This was frustrating for both mothers and midwives, who knew that they could receive ongoing responsible care if only the midwives were allowed to practise in an environment with ready access to the technology the mother might require.

By the 1980s, midwives and their supporters were agitating for a better understanding and acceptance of midwifery by the Canadian public, the medical profession and governments. In an effort to change public opinion and government policy, midwifery advocates were organizing and attending conferences and rallies and writing books in support of the profession. But some of the surprising catalysts for midwifery legislation were high-profile legal challenges: inquests and investigations of midwives' abilities and choices following the deaths of babies. In Ontario in 1982 and 1985, formal legal challenges of midwifery care were undertaken during coroners' inquests into baby deaths. In British Columbia during the 1980s, several highly publicized court cases involving baby deaths (one resulted in an inquiry in 1986 and one in an inquest in 1988), served to expose the controversies swirling around midwifery and contributed to recommendations that midwifery be legislated and supported by government. In 1981 in

Alberta, doctors were banned from attending homebirths by their college. Parents and practitioners alike were outraged that their access to choice in birth was being limited.

Legal challenges were a galvanizing force for midwives, clients and their supporters. Advocates of midwifery raised money to pay the legal fees for challenges, prepared briefs and sent out press releases in an effort to inform the courts and the public about their experience of midwifery, which involved compassionate, informed care; satisfied, confident clients; and healthy breastfed babies.

**Midwifery is essential**

Even today the midwife attends two-thirds of all births in the world. She is the basic caregiver for maternity care services in every single European country. And in the European countries with the lowest infant mortality rates (all lower than the United States, which ranks an embarrassing 21st in infant mortality), the midwife is the senior person attending at 75 percent of all births, whether the birth occurs in a hospital, a clinic or the home. It is, therefore, an incredible enigma that women within the United States and Canada can be denied the services of a midwife when the rest of the world considers midwifery to be an essential and basic service.

—*Marsden Wagner, M.D., Former Director of Women's and Children's Health, World Health Organization (WHO)*

Most midwives and midwifery clients supported a move to regulated midwifery. But some women had serious concerns that midwifery would become institutionalized and lose its egalitarian and woman-centred roots. It became clear that if the new midwifery was to reflect any of the values and beliefs that had come to define midwifery in Canada, then midwives would have to be instrumental in its design and implementation.

Making this decision to become part of the legislated and publicly funded health care system was difficult for many, and in some areas the conflict is still very much alive. Some women who used to call themselves midwives now quietly practise as "traditional birth attendants," preferring to work outside the system, instead of complying with set standards of care that they feel compromise their clients' experience.

Those midwives who embraced the move to legislation decided to become architects of the new system. In 1993, Ontario became the first province to legislate and fund midwifery, and the first registered midwives began practising in 1994. The first graduates from the Ontario Midwifery Education Program started practising in 1996. British Columbia followed with registration of midwives in 1998. Quebec registered midwives in a pilot project in 1994, which was followed with province-wide registration in 1999.

The move toward greater access to midwifery service seems slow or inevitable, depending on your perspective. But as more consumers experience midwifery care, and the understanding of midwifery as a profession and a service grows, so does the demand.

## Today's Midwifery

Since Ontario was the first province to implement midwifery legislation, the model of care has provided something of a template for other areas. The Ontario model is based on the principles of continuity of care, informed choice and choice of birthplace. Midwives generally work together in group practices, and women get to know at least two midwives during their care. Midwives spend time developing relationships with women and are available 24 hours a day, seven days a week. Women are active decision-makers in the care they receive and are expected to take responsibility for their choices. In Ontario, choice of birth place involves choosing between home and hospital. Other provinces with midwifery legislation have much in common with Ontario's model, but there are variations from province to province. A breakdown by province or territory follows later in this chapter.

Canadian midwifery meets the international standards as defined by the World Health Organization. Canadian midwifery principles and practice have also been examined with favourable results by makers of midwifery policy in countries such as Holland and Sweden, which have stellar reputations for midwifery care. Many Canadian midwives engage in regular ongoing professional development and discussion with their colleagues in other countries. Midwifery in Canada has come a long way in the past decade. Ten years ago there was no midwifery legislation, yet today Canadian midwifery has an international reputation for excellence in education and practice.

**Definition of the midwife—World Health Organization**

A midwife is a person who, having been regularly admitted to a midwifery educational programme, duly recognised in the country in which it is located, has successfully completed the prescribed course of studies in midwifery and has acquired the requisite qualifications to be registered and/or legally licensed to practise midwifery.

She must be able to give the necessary supervision, care and advice to women during pregnancy, labour and the postpartum period, to conduct deliveries on her own responsibility and to care for the newborn and the infant. This care includes preventative measures, the detection of abnormal conditions in mother and child, the procurement of medical assistance and the execution of emergency measures in the absence of medical help. She has an important task in health counselling and education, not only for the women, but also within the family and the community. The work should involve antenatal education and preparation for parenthood and extends to certain areas of gynaecology, family planning and child care. She may practise in hospitals, clinics, health units, domiciliary conditions or in any other service.

*Jointly developed by the International Confederation of Midwives*
*and the International Federation of Gynaecology and Obstetrics, 1972*

Although midwives are in great demand almost everywhere they practise, the number of babies caught by Canadian midwives is only a handful compared to countries with a more established midwifery system. In comparison to that in the 75 percent of the world's babies caught by midwives, in British Columbia less than 7 percent of babies were born with the help of 66 midwives in 2000. In the same year in Ontario, only about 4.5 percent of babies were born to women under the care of the province's 200 registered midwives.

Recently, when Miranda sat in on a first-year Women's Studies lecture at Carleton University, she was amazed that only one of the dozens of students in attendance knew that midwifery in Ontario is paid for by the government. Even in areas where midwifery has been legislated and funded for several years, in hospitals where midwives catch babies on a daily basis, a woman may have to explain repeatedly that there is no obstetrician's name on her test requisition form because the midwife is her primary caregiver. Understanding of midwifery has a long way to go. However, there are great success stories, too, of collaborative efforts among medical personnel and effective educational campaigns. For example, in a hospital-based birth centre in Winnipeg, all forms and documents contain references to the "doctor or midwife." In many areas, midwives report very positive experiences in working with hospital staff.

While much of the old stigma and misinformation still lingers around the word *midwifery*, another reason for confusion is that midwifery is not yet legislated in all provinces or territories. In some places, legislation has been accompanied by funding; in others, this is not the case. Almost every legislated area offers a choice of birth place, with the exception of Quebec. As of 2002, Quebec midwives were not officially practising within the home and were restricted to practising midwifery in birth centres. Even in areas where midwifery is not legislated, there may be active pockets of midwifery with very good standards of care. What seems consistent across the country is a commitment to a kind of care that puts the woman at the centre and responds to her wishes and needs, as well as promoting a birth free of unnecessary interventions.

## Midwifery in Your Province or Territory

In almost every province with legislated midwifery, there are provincial colleges that act as the regulating body. The colleges provide midwives with their registration. There are also provincial associations that represent midwives as a professional body, providing professional development, public relations and lobbying on their behalf. Finally, in a growing number of provinces there are midwifery education programs that set and deliver curricula at the university level. Some provinces have midwifery legislation, some have funding and some offer choice of birth place—and some have all three elements. In other areas, there may be active midwifery practices not yet recognized by provincial legislation.

| Province | Legislated | Funded | Fee for Service | Home/Hospital/ Birth Centre | Education Program |
|---|---|---|---|---|---|
| Alberta | Yes | No | Yes | Home/Hospital/ Birth Centre | No |
| British Columbia | Yes | Yes | No | Home/Hospital | Yes |
| Manitoba | Yes | Yes | No | Home/Hospital | No |
| Newfoundland and Labrador | No | No | No | Hospital (remote areas only) | No |
| New Brunswick | No | No | Yes | Home | No |
| Northwest Territories | No | No | Yes | Home | No |
| Nova Scotia | No | No | Yes | Home | No |
| Nunavut | Partially (one pilot project in 2002) | Partially | No | Birth Centre (only in Rankin Inlet) | No |
| Ontario | Yes | Yes | No | Home/Hospital | Yes |
| Prince Edward Island | No | No | Yes | Home | No |
| Quebec | Yes | Yes | No | Birth Centre | Yes |
| Saskatchewan | Yes | No | Yes | Home | No |
| Yukon | No | No | Yes | Home | No |

*Alberta*

In Alberta, midwives have been government-regulated health practitioners since 1998. However, at this time they are not funded. This means that if

Albertan women choose midwifery care they pay a fee, set at $2500 in 2002.

A registered midwife in Alberta can provide all prenatal, labour, birth and postpartum care. Midwives in Alberta may prescribe medications, order diagnostic tests, and admit clients to hospital. Midwives can attend labouring women either at their home or in the hospital. In Calgary, midwives can also offer their clients the use of a private free-standing birth centre. Additional fees (around $500) are paid directly to the birth centre for this service.

There are currently between 20 and 30 midwives practising in about six locations in Alberta.

Alberta does not yet have a college that registers midwives. Instead, the Midwifery Health Disciplines Committee, which is funded and governed by Alberta Health and Wellness, assesses midwives' qualifications and issues registration. The Association of Alberta Midwives promotes and supports midwifery. Alberta is also home to a very strong and organized consumer movement. Two consumer magazines that support midwifery and homebirth are published in Alberta. *Birthing* is published in Calgary and *Birth Issues* in Edmonton. See the appendix for information about where to find these periodicals.

Clients who choose midwifery in Alberta tend to be very motivated and to recognize the value of a service for which they pay directly. Women and their families are drawn to the service by the type of care that midwives provide and also by the homebirth option. Many of the Alberta midwives say that the majority of their homebirth clients choose to birth in water.

Funding for midwifery in Alberta is still being discussed. Some midwives and mothers hope that the government will make a commitment soon. Others worry that funding midwifery services will compromise midwives' autonomy.

### British Columbia

Midwives in British Columbia have been legislated and funded by the province since 1998. Midwives in this province may order appropriate diagnostic tests, such as blood work and ultrasound examinations. They can also order and administer certain medications used by some women during pregnancy and childbirth. Midwives can attend mothers either at home or in hospital.

There are more than 65 registered midwives practising in approximately 30 different cities and towns in B.C.

A college of midwives provides registration and governs the policies and practices of the profession. There is also an association that offers professional support and public education about the role of midwives. A midwifery education program has been implemented at the University of British Columbia. The consumer group in B.C. is affiliated with the Association for the Improvement of Maternity Services (AIMS). AIMS is a consumer organization based in the United Kingdom that has international chapters, including one in British Columbia. AIMS has replaced British Columbia's Midwifery Task Force, which was the stakeholder group advocating for legislated and funded midwifery in the province.

Although B.C. has the second highest number of midwives in the country, demand far exceeds supply. Each midwife provides care to 40 women every year; with more than 40,000 annual births in the province, only a small number of women currently have access to midwives. Midwifery practices fill up quickly so it is advisable for women to call in the early stages of their pregnancies in order to be ensured a place in midwifery care.

### Manitoba

Midwifery has been regulated and funded in Manitoba since 2000. Midwives practise as employees of the regional health authorities, and their availability depends on the willingness of the local health authority to apply for funding to employ them. Midwives catch babies at home and in hospital. Midwives may order all of the tests and perform all of the assessment and diagnostics necessary for the complete care of pregnant women and newborn babies.

Approximately 25 midwives (in 2002) practise in five regional health authority catchment areas. The catchment areas are fairly strict; women who live outside the prescribed geographic boundaries will not be able to see the midwives who practise there. The majority of Manitoba's practising midwives are concentrated in Winnipeg.

There is both a college and an Association of Manitoba Midwives, but these organizations are still in their infancy. Much of the profession's focus has been on setting up service and integrating midwifery into the public health care system.

Midwives currently practising in Manitoba received their training in a variety of places and through different methods, including self-study, apprenticeship, education programs in other provinces, and clinical placements in other countries. All midwives who are practising either have registration in another province or were part of the training and assessment program run by the province to register midwives.

A strong homebirth community has existed in Manitoba for years, and the incidence of water labour and birth is also quite high in this province. One practice estimated that 70 percent of births took place in water.

Midwives practise in health care clinics or in facilities owned by the regional health authority. This situation in which midwives share space with other, more established health care professionals is unusual in Canadian midwifery practice.


### New Brunswick

In New Brunswick midwifery is not regulated or publicly funded. Nor is there an organized consumer group. Occasionally, fee-for-service homebirth midwives can be found.


### Newfoundland and Labrador

Newfoundland and Labrador was the last province to eliminate midwifery, and it has been one of the most resistant to its revival. Midwives served the far-flung communities for years, but once funded medical care was implemented in the province, women opted for paid maternity services. The last licence to practise midwifery was issued in 1963. Although midwifery has never been illegal in Newfoundland, there is no longer a mechanism for issuing credentials to qualified practitioners, and it has been impossible to get a licence since 1963.

In particularly remote areas of the province, hospital labour floors are staffed by nurse-midwives. They do not necessarily provide continuity of care and may only practise in a hospital setting.

However, there is a provincial organization for midwives. The Newfoundland and Labrador Midwives Association holds meetings and issues four newsletters a year. Supporters of midwifery lobby policy makers to promote the profession. But until legislation is passed, there will be few opportunities for midwives to thrive in Newfoundland and Labrador.

### Northwest Territories

Midwifery in the Northwest Territories is not regulated or funded. Most women must leave their communities at 36 to 38 weeks in order to give birth at larger hospitals, because there are no community-based options. Some public support exists for community-based birthing, but there is little accompanying support from the health care system.

There are two practising midwives (both registered in other provinces) who provide fee-for-service care in Fort Smith. These midwives practise a model of care similar to that found elsewhere in Canada.

The midwives of the Northwest Territories are currently trying to create a midwives association for the NWT and Nunavut.

### Nova Scotia

Midwifery is not funded or legislated in Nova Scotia, but there are currently three midwives who provide prenatal, labour and postpartum care for women who give birth at home. These midwives are based in Halifax and Wolfville, but they have been known to travel across the province—and even to other under-serviced provinces—to aid women committed to homebirth. Their clients arrange to see a doctor for tests and for any necessary medications, and as a pre-emptive measure in case complications arise during their homebirth and they need to go to hospital. Despite the fact that the midwives have no privileges at the hospitals, they report relatively good relations with the medical teams they encounter. Midwives' fees are paid on a sliding scale according to the client's income.

The Midwifery Coalition of Nova Scotia has been active for more than 20 years. This organization has a substantial paid membership. It issues a regular newsletter and brings in internationally known speakers. Despite its efforts, however, midwifery legislation has failed to capture the interest of the government in power long enough to bring about legislative change.

### Nunavut

The Nunavut Department of Health and Social Services funds a pilot midwifery project at a birth centre in Rankin Inlet. However, there is no official body to register midwives in Nunavut. In order to practise there, a midwife must have registration in her home province or country of origin. In addition to the Rankin Inlet birth centre there are approximately 20 community health nurses (CHNs) with midwifery qualifications working in the territory.

Midwives in Rankin Inlet provide care in much the same manner as their counterparts in other areas of Canada. There are no midwives who speak Inuktitut, but there is a movement afoot to establish a community-based midwifery education program.

### Ontario

Midwifery in Ontario is both legislated and funded. Registered midwives have been providing care since 1994. Their clients may give birth at home or in hospital, and the midwives handle all stages of care, from prenatal through to six weeks postpartum. Tests, assessments and provision of some prescriptions all fall within their scope of practice. Midwives in Ontario, like their counterparts elsewhere, provide care to women experiencing a normal pregnancy. However, they can consult with other health care providers and sometimes share care with them should the need arise.

By 2002, there were 250 registered midwives providing care in more than 30 cities and towns across Ontario.

The Association of Ontario Midwives (AOM) provides professional development and lobbying support. The AOM has published a journal for several years, which evolved in 2002 into a national publication in co-operation with the Canadian Association of Midwives. The Ontario College of Midwives governs the profession and issues registration. The Midwifery Education Program, which was established in 1993 and graduated its first class in 1996, offers a degree-granting program at three Ontario universities. The Ontario college also evaluates the skills and education of midwives who come to Ontario from other countries through a process called the Prior Learning and Education Assessment (PLEA). Once these women meet Ontario standards, they become registered midwives.

### Prince Edward Island

There is no legislation or funding for midwifery services in Prince Edward Island. As of 2002 there are no practising midwives in the province who provide homebirth on a fee-for-service basis. The Prince Edward Island Midwives Association (PEIMA) is lobbying the local government to integrate midwifery into the health care system.

### Quebec

The midwifery profession became fully legal and funded in Quebec in 1999. Midwives in this province currently practise only in free-standing birth centres, although homebirth is expected to become an option in the future. All birth centres are associated with local community health centres. In other ways, the midwifery model in Quebec resembles that of other provinces.

Midwives provide continuous care throughout the prenatal, labour and postpartum periods. Tests and diagnostics normally associated with pregnancy fall within their scope of practice.

There are approximately 55 midwives currently working in seven birthing centres in six cities and towns scattered throughout Quebec. In the Northern Quebec communities of Puvurnituq and Inukjuak, birth centres provide the opportunity for the largely Inuit population to stay close to their home community for prenatal and postpartum care, as well as for the birth itself. The centre is staffed primarily by Inuit midwives, who receive their training in the community.

As in other provinces there is an association that provides midwives with professional support, and a college that issues licences and sets standards of practice. A midwifery education program is also offered at the University of Quebec in Trois Rivières.

Each birth centre has a staff of three to eight midwives, who work as individuals as well as part of a team. Birth centres also employ birth assistants, who assist during labours. These assistants provide food and supplementary care to midwives and clients. Birth assistants, or *aides-natales* also help clients during the postpartum period and offer breastfeeding support. Each birth centre is a unique environment, decorated with care to create a home-like atmospehere. Each centre has a stock of homeopathic remedies and birth aids, which include tubs for labour and birth. Intravenous supplements can also be used at birthing centres. In the event that a woman requires a transfer to hospital, the midwife must transfer her care to a physician. Depending on the location, the physician will then allow the midwife a degree of participation: in some cases midwives catch their clients' babies even after they are transferred; in others they simply provide ongoing emotional support.

*Saskatchewan*

The Saskatchewan government passed the *Midwifery Act* in 1999 allowing regulated midwives to practise, but it has made no commitment to funding. There is a Midwives Association of Saskatchewan and two consumer support groups, one in Saskatoon and one in Regina.

*Yukon*

It is possible, on a limited scale, to find a midwife who runs a fee-for-service practice. Though the government has considered legislating and funding midwifery, it has made no commitments yet.

## The Outlook for Canadian Midwifery

Despite the gains the midwifery profession has made in the past 10 years, it still faces many challenges. Some provinces are struggling for funding and others for legitimacy. Many doctors and nurses now consider midwives colleagues and may recommend midwifery care to their patients or choose it for their own births. However, in some communities, individual health care professionals may feel hesitant or even hostile about midwifery, the women who practise it and their clients. Access to midwifery training is an issue for women who live outside major centres where education programs are based, or in provinces with no midwifery education programs at all. First Nations and Inuit midwives still face great challenges around training and regulation.

Advocates fight for funding on a yearly basis, even in provinces where midwifery has been established for years. Malpractice insurance remains one of the most difficult issues for midwives and for health care ministries; the premiums increase exponentially, at one time jumping by more than 400 percent in a single year.

The consumer movement, so integral to the formation of professional midwifery, remains strong in some parts of the country, while in others, having slept through the post-legislation years, it is waking up to the new issues of the day.

In some areas, midwives' increasing comfort with medical technology is causing concern. For example, will allowing midwives to administer epidurals change the core values of midwifery or will it support choice and continuity of care? Will schools continue to graduate midwives who are comfortable with homebirth, the roots of midwifery, and who are committed to care that is truly woman-centred?

A poster we spotted in practices around Toronto aptly proclaimed midwifery to be "the oldest and newest profession." Rich in history and with a solid philosophical stance, Canadian midwifery is still defining itself, one mother at a time.

## ◎ If You Want to Read More . . .

*Birth by Design: Pregnancy, Maternity Care, and Midwifery in North America and Europe*, by Raymond Devries, *et al*. (New York: Routledge, 2001).

*Birth Reborn*, by Dr. Michael Odent (New York: Random House, 1984).

*The Experience of Childbirth* (5th ed.), by Sheila Kitzinger ( Harmondsworth: Penguin, 1987).

*Immaculate Deception II: Myth Magic and Birth*, by Suzanne Arms (Berkeley, California: Celestial Arts, 1994).

*Birth Without Violence: Revised Edition of the Classic*, by Frederick Leboyer (Rochester, Vermont: Inner Traditions International, 2002).

*In Labor: Women and Power in the Birthplace*, by Barbara Katz Rothman (New York: Norton, 1991).

*The Midwife Challenge*, by Sheila Kitzinger (ed.) (London: Pandora Press, 1991).

*Midwifery Is Catching*, by Eleanor Barrington (Toronto: NC Press Limited, 1985).

*The New Midwifery: Reflections on Renaissance and Regulation*, by Farah M. Shroff (ed.) (Toronto: Women's Press, 1997).

*Spiritual Midwifery* (3rd ed.), by Ina May Gaskin (Summertown, Tennessee: The Book Publishing Company, 1990).

*Trials of Labour: The Re-emergence of Midwifery*, by Brian Burtch (Montreal and Kingston: McGill–Queen's University Press, 1994).

*Witches, Midwives, and Nurses: A History of Women Healers* by Barbara Ehrenreich and Deirdre English (New York: The Feminist Press, 1973).

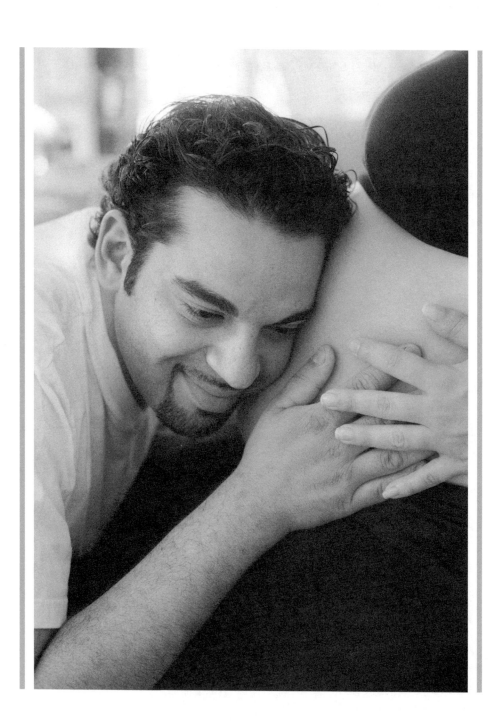

## Three

# Building Support for Your Choice:
## Talking about Myths and Reality

In some communities, women routinely choose midwives, having been encouraged to do so by family, friends or colleagues who have made the same choice. But in most places and social circles in Canada, a woman who chooses midwifery care is making a decision that stands out.

Deciding who will care for you and your baby is among the most personal and private decisions you will make. For us, those decisions were also among the most *important* we made: they influenced our feelings about ourselves, our babies and our growing families long after the babies were born.

Of course, this is your body and your baby. But very few people act entirely independently. Having a baby is a big deal, and most of us would prefer that someone close to us understand, and even applaud, our decisions.

When choosing your care, in addition to reflecting on your own beliefs, you will probably consider the opinions of the people who mean the most to you: your partner, parents and close friends. How they feel about you and the way they communicate this to you could matter a great deal, particularly during pregnancy when you may feel more vulnerable than usual.

If you are in a relationship, you and your mate will probably want to approach the pregnancy, birth and your child's life as partners. But if you are sold on midwifery care and your partner has fears or reservations about it, this difference of opinion may create a rift at a time when you want to be a team. It may not be enough to have your partner merely accept your choices, although we certainly know women who have done this with some success. The ideal situation is for both of you to embrace your decisions about care. This doesn't mean you will instantly share the same ideas about care and the birth itself, but the ability to share your questions and eventually your decisions is invaluable.

### A father adjusts to the idea of midwifery

I grew up in a working-class neighbourhood with working-class parents who gave me working-class ideals. I went to church every Sunday, Cubs on Tuesdays and Ukrainian dance classes on Saturdays. I was brought up to be a conformist. I was taught not to argue with my teachers or question authority. Drawing attention to myself was frowned upon. The mould was set early and I learned my lessons well.

When my wife Lorraine and I found out that we were expecting, we were understandably ecstatic. Men of the nineties had evolved into creatures who participated in the child-rearing process. They changed diapers, applied zinc oxide to rashes, cleaned up vomit and washed babies' clothing in separate loads with Ivory Snow. I was ready and eager to perform tasks that my father never would have dreamed of doing.

Well, you can imagine my horror when Lorraine suggested that we use a midwife to deliver our baby. I was even more shocked when she said she wanted to have the baby at home! If it was good enough for my mother to go to the hospital, be knocked out and given her child hours later after awaking from a drug-induced stupor, then, by golly, it was good enough for my wife. Honestly! What if there was an emergency? My gosh, midwives aren't even doctors. More like witch doctors!

Lorraine was adamant, though, and she made an appointment with a practice near our home. After the initial shock, I remembered that I am a man of the nineties. Compassionate, caring, open-minded. We'd go to see the midwife and I'd reserve judgement until after the meeting.

I was thoroughly impressed with our prospective midwife. She answered all our questions effectively and professionally—and believe me, there were many. I got a strong sense of the compassion and dedication this midwife brought to her profession. These women were obviously trained professionals. And we would have an added bonus of a second certified midwife with us, not to mention a student who

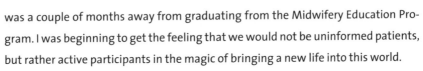

was a couple of months away from graduating from the Midwifery Education Program. I was beginning to get the feeling that we would not be uninformed patients, but rather active participants in the magic of bringing a new life into this world.

—*Russ, father of two*

Parents, your partners' parents, siblings and close friends may all have strong opinions about your care. If you are lucky, their opinions and approaches may complement yours. But if, in choosing your care, you find yourself taking an alternative stance from the other people in your support circle, you may begin to wonder how much you want to be seen as a pioneer.

If this is your first child, you also may be astonished to find that everyone from the woman at the community centre to the man in front of you at the checkout has something to say about motherhood and how it's supposed to go. Get ready. This is only the beginning. People seem to have an irrepressible need to comment on your parenting choices as well as your belly size. Learning to determine your own way, and then to stand up for it, will probably become a big part of your new role as a mother.

Some women also report opposition from their regular health care provider. Some doctors and nurses recommend midwives, but others try to steer women away from the midwifery option, suggesting that it is not a safe choice, or that the woman in question is a poor candidate for midwifery care.

There will always be people who simply oppose an idea because it is not the way things are usually done. But many people who object to midwifery care do so because of a lack of information or an abundance of misinformation. If you encounter opposition from people who matter to you, it may help you to familiarize yourself with some of the myths that continue to haunt midwifery and some of the common arguments against opting for midwifery care.

## Midwifery Myths and Reality

**Myth:** To have a midwife, you must choose a homebirth.

**Reality:** Midwives attempt to give their clients a choice of birth place: depending on where you live, this may be home, hospital or birth centre. Arguments against midwifery are often arguments against homebirth. If you are considering a homebirth and are dealing with your own misgivings or others', see Chapter 6, where we deal with homebirth options.

**Myth:** Midwives will try anything to get you to birth at home.

**Reality:** Midwifery in Canada is governed by the principle of informed choice: midwives provide the information, you make the choice. Midwives in many parts of Canada attend women labouring in hospital or a birth centre as well as at home. If you choose a midwife who practises in more than one location, then you have the opportunity to give birth in either place. This is your baby's birth, not the midwives', and they will support your choice.

Midwives remain the only professionals trained and willing to attend women who choose to have their babies at home. So you will hear about the homebirth option and have the opportunity to consider whether it would be right for you.

**Myth:** Women who choose midwives care more about the experience than the baby.

**Reality:** The work that midwives do to help mothers through the birth experience has repeatedly been shown to have a positive impact on the mother's physical and emotional health, as well as the baby's. Women who feel supported during labour and who are not subjected to unnecessary interventions report less pain and less "eventful" births, which makes it easier for their babies to be born strong and alert. The attention midwives pay to a woman's emotional health has a strong impact on her physical health.

**Myth:** Women choose midwives because they don't understand the risks involved in birth.

**Reality:** Because midwives offer women a great deal of information so they can make decisions about everything from nutrition to place of birth to breastfeeding, midwifery clients may be better informed than their counterparts, who may choose a style of care in which many decisions are made for them. Among the things that midwifery clients know or will learn is that research shows midwifery has equally good results for the health of mothers and newborns when compared with care provided by physicians.

### Gaining confidence

Our midwife helped give us a lot of confidence in what we were doing. . . . Generally I think the idea is that the woman is in control of the birth, responsible for the birth, and is able to do it. The woman should believe in herself as the most important person present, rather than the doctors being in control and telling her when to sit up or sit down. I think a lot of women feel insecure or lack the confidence in themselves that they need for giving birth. The midwives work from the initial assumption that a woman is able to give birth to a child and has all the natural functions necessary to do so. And with the confidence and understanding of how the mechanisms work, there really shouldn't be a problem.

*Kevin, father of one*

**Myth:** There is no place for men in midwifery care.

**Reality:** Midwives acknowledge birthing as women's work. Who wouldn't? But that doesn't mean they believe that supporting a woman in labour is a job only for women. Midwives recognize and encourage the participation of the important people in your life—whoever they may be. Many fathers point out that the midwives provided *them* with great care, as well as looking after the mother and baby.

**Joel catches his son**

Our biggest request was that my husband Joel would be able to deliver. As a paramedic he'd been trained in emergency deliveries and was eager to experience birth first-hand—especially that of his own child. With our first we had hoped he could catch, but our wishes were not carried through since we didn't have a chance to go over our birth plan with the doctor and didn't feel comfortable requesting this during the delivery. For our second child, our midwife was thrilled with the idea, and we figured Joel would just be able to catch, but in the end our midwife helped deliver our son into his bare hands. The experience was an incredible one, which my husband and I will cherish forever. Joel was crying so hard he could barely see to cut the cord.

—*Melanie, mother of two*

**Myth:** "You can't have a midwife. You're high-risk."
**Reality:** Maybe you are. Women who truly have a high risk of complications are not attended by midwives. However, the phrase "high-risk pregnancy" has been used to describe all kinds of circumstances, from having a baby after age 35, to a petite woman's first pregnancy, to women trying for a vaginal birth after a C-section. Midwives attend women with a wide variety of histories and experiences, and they will not take on clients for whom they cannot provide optimal care. Though some conditions may restrict your choice of birth place—for example, having twins—you may still be able to choose midwives as your caregivers for a hospital birth. Consult with a midwife before counting yourself out of midwifery care.

**Myth:** Midwives are for women who can handle pain or who have easy labours.
**Reality:** A minuscule number of women report that their midwife-assisted births were not painful. Shocking, yet true. But almost all women experience pain during labour. While midwives can't eliminate the pain, they are fantastic at helping women manage it without medical interventions. We have met

many women who were particularly frightened about labour pain and who sought midwifery care for just this reason. During labour, if you feel you cannot continue without pain relief, midwives will arrange to get the drugs you need. Also, if the midwives feel that pain relief will help your labour to progress (so that you can avoid further interventions such as a C-section), they will recommend and facilitate the use of pain-relieving drugs.

**Myth:** Midwives don't let you have drugs.

**Reality:** Midwives are advocates of birth without unnecessary interventions, and in most cases this includes elements that have become standard in medicalized birth, such as the routine use of episiotomies and epidurals, and the requirement that labouring mothers stay in bed. However, midwives also know how to determine when an intervention is appropriate for the mother or the infant, and will not deny you drugs or an epidural if you want them. But it is important to remember that midwives can help women give birth in such a way that they won't necessarily need drugs or any other intervention.

**Myth:** Midwives force you to sip herbal tea and chant.

**Reality:** Midwives often know about natural remedies for the discomforts of pregnancy and postpartum. They may suggest herbs for postpartum baths, natural treatments for sore breasts, or teas and vitamins for things like increasing a mother's milk supply. Midwives may also help women use their voices more effectively to facilitate labour, suggest unconventional positions for labouring and advise women to condition the perineal area before birth with stretches and massages. It is possible that they will tell you about natural methods of encouraging labour, such as increasing sexual activity. They will also inform you about conventional medical approaches. You are no more obligated to accept these alternative options than you are to embrace diagnostic testing or a particular place of birth. The choice is yours.

**Myth:** Midwives are expensive.

**Reality:** In most areas where midwifery is legislated, funding is provided through the health care system. If you live in a province that has midwifery legislation but no funding, however, you will have to pay for your own care. A case in point is Alberta, where midwives have agreed to charge the same amount for each birth. As of 2002 that amount was a $2500 flat fee. A birth centre in Calgary charges an additional $500 for the use of its facilities. In a province like Nova Scotia, which has neither legislation nor funding, midwives charge for their services on a sliding scale according to their clients' income. The bill may run from $800 to just under $2000.

**Myth:** You can't get any tests if you have midwives.

**Reality:** In areas where midwifery is legislated, midwives can order a wide range of tests, covering everything you are likely to need during pregnancy. Where midwifery is not legislated, midwives can't order tests. However, women in these areas usually choose to see a doctor periodically, partly to get blood work done or to order tests such as ultrasounds or amniocentesis. Midwives who practise in these areas may be able to recommend a doctor who understands your choice to use midwives and who will provide supportive care.

**Myth:** Midwives are less experienced than doctors or nurses.

**Reality:** Midwives are often referred to as "experts in normal birth." They don't set broken bones, but they do know how to catch babies. Midwives are experts in the entire birth process. Doctors may deliver as many as eight babies in one busy night shift; full-time midwives in Ontario attend eight births per month but provide care throughout the entire act of labour. Still, it is not uncommon to encounter midwives with long careers who have caught well over a thousand babies.

**Myth:** Midwives and doctors don't respect each other.

**Reality:** Some doctors still question the idea of midwifery as a profession. Even in hospitals where midwives and doctors practise just down the hall from one another, doctors can still misunderstand the work midwives do. However, many, many doctors are advocates of midwifery and routinely suggest it as an option to their patients. Some doctors are even clients themselves. Today, in many instances, midwives and doctors practise as colleagues and respect and acknowledge one another's separate skills.

### Common ideals

I made an appointment to ask my GP what she thought of midwives. When she found out which midwife I had seen, she said: "That's funny, that's my midwife." If my own GP was choosing a midwife, why shouldn't I?

*–Kira, mother of one*

**Myth:** "If I (my sister/my wife) had had a midwife, the baby would have died."

**Reality:** This statement is tricky, because it's so personal, but we have included it because we hear it often. Sometimes this argument comes from people who do not recognize that many of the difficult situations they have experienced or heard about—like excessive bleeding after the baby is born, or babies who needed resuscitation—are situations that midwives are trained to handle. Midwives are not able to perform C-sections, which are sometimes required for both mother and child, but they have access to someone who can. Midwives have skills that allow them to cover a variety of situations, and they also monitor how a birth is progressing so that they can get you the help of a doctor at a hospital if you need it.

**Myth:** Midwives won't do you any good if you have a C-section.

**Reality:** Studies from Canada and abroad show that midwifery clients are less likely to have a C-section than mothers who opt for a physician-assisted birth. To be fair, the midwives' numbers are stacked in favour of "natural" birth because midwives do not specialize in high-risk clients. However, midwifery clients do sometimes have labours that develop in such a way that a C-section is required. Some of the most ardent supporters of midwifery care are those women whose midwives held their hands and explained the procedure while the medical team concentrated on the surgery they required.

### C-section with midwife support

Around 11 P.M., they prepped me for the C-section. The nurses got a chair and put it outside the door for Guy to sit on. He wasn't allowed to come in with me, because I would be under general anesthetic. I remember him sitting there looking forlorn.

They wheeled me into an operating room, lifted me onto a table, and started strapping me down to it. At that point it felt like chaos. There were really bright lights, and it seemed to me there were people all over the place. The doctor stood behind me, and I couldn't see his face, but he was talking to me, and he was about to put me under. I remember turning to my midwife and saying, "Am I going to be O.K.? Is everything going to be O.K.?" And she held my hand. That was so important to me, because Guy couldn't be with me, and it was just terrifying, overwhelming. My midwife explained that both my midwives would be there; she was going to be watching me, and the other midwife was going to watch the baby, so they would have an eye on each of us the whole time.

Then the anesthesiologist put the mask on my face. It was really tight and I thought, "Oh, my God, I'm suffocating." But the last thing I remember feeling was my midwife's hand holding mine. And I knew that everything would be all right, because she was there.

The next thing I remember were voices around me. I guess my eyelids were fluttering because I heard the voices say, "She's waking up." Then I heard Guy say in French, "It's a little girl." I still couldn't open my eyes but I felt myself smile; it just felt so right. I remember opening my eyes, and seeing Guy standing there holding her. Then I passed out again.

Later Guy told me he heard our baby when she came out; the next thing he saw was a nurse go with her into another room, then he saw that the midwife was with her, and he could go be with the baby and the midwife right away. I think they were a comfort to him, too.

After I woke up, the midwives stayed with me for quite a while. They put my baby to my breast and she started nursing right away. I remember counting my blessings at that point.

Over the next few days, I was a bit traumatized by this whole thing. But my midwives kept visiting while I cried and talked to them about it. I was worrying that my condition [HELLP Syndrome] was going to affect me permanently, that maybe I'd hold it against my daughter, Isabel, and it would taint my relationship with her. But they talked me through all of it.

When I look back, I thank God for the health care system that we have. I was lucky to have good medical care when I needed it. But most of all, I felt lucky to have my midwives there the whole time. I would have felt so freaked out without them, but I could always get reassurance from them or further clarification when I didn't understand something. Just having my midwife hold my hand at that moment in surgery was so important.

Afterwards, I said to the doctor, "Does this condition mean I need to have obstetric care next time?" And he said, "No, it won't make a difference."

Now I tell everyone: If something goes wrong, your midwives will transfer you to the care you need, but you'll be luckier than any other person in that situation; you'll be with health care professionals who really know you and can attend to your needs when all the other medical staff are too busy.

—*Barb, mother of one*

**Myth:** Midwives don't know how to deal with problems in pregnancy and birth.

**Reality:** Midwives are specialists in normal birth, but that does not mean they are unfamiliar with identifying complications that may arise. If you or your baby develop a condition that requires help that is beyond their scope of practice, midwives will consult with a physician who can help decide what action to take to give you the best care possible.

**Myth:** Once you're in labour, you won't care who's there.

**Reality:** This is a very common belief, but not among women who've had midwives. In the rush and chaos of a busy labour and delivery floor, where all the doctors and nurses are strangers to you, it is possible for them to help you to get that baby out of your body without your developing any strong feelings about the other people in the room. However, women who have had babies with midwives usually remember their reassuring and familiar presence as being integral to the labour, birth and first few hours with their new babies.

**Myth:** Women who have midwives go home from the hospital too soon, so their babies are at risk.

**Reality:** Mothers and babies who are attended by midwives in the hospital are often discharged a few hours after the birth. Unlike those women who are discharged early after being cared for only by hospital personnel, mothers who choose midwives will be visited at home within 24 hours and on many other days until the baby is several weeks old. In addition, they'll be able to get in touch with their midwife, night or day, by telephone until their baby is at least six weeks old.

**Mothering the mother**

Once we came home, our midwife continued to provide unending support. She demonstrated the true picture of mothering the mother. She always made us feel looked after and taken care of.

—*Jacqueline, mother of four*

## Working Through Opposition

Fortunately, many people are able to understand the importance of midwifery care once they have a personal encounter with it. We've come across numerous people who confess they once had a knee-jerk reaction to the idea of midwifery care, but who are now avid supporters of midwives and families who choose them. These converts include medical personnel, journalists and policy-makers, as well as midwifery clients and their extended families.

**One dad's first reaction to midwives**

I don't want my baby delivered by a coven of witches.

*—Jeff, now a proud father*
*of two children caught by midwives*

Many mothers cope with criticism by turning a deaf ear to it, while others choose to re-educate their critics. How much you want to be an educational force is up to you. You may not feel particularly enthusiastic about explaining your choice while your pregnancy and your plans for your baby consume your brain and body. Other people enjoy sharing their enthusiasm for their care with even the most reluctant friends and family.

So how can you help bring your circle of supporters along so that they can embrace the choices you've made and help you through your pregnancy, birth and life with a new baby? You can lend them videos and books (such as this one or any from the recommended reading list), and refer them to informative sites on the Internet. But by far the most reassuring approach is to talk to women who've chosen midwives, or, better yet, with the midwives themselves. It seems that for most people, from other health care workers to nervous grandmothers, just meeting a midwife makes all the difference.

Obviously, it is not practical for you to traipse through the midwives' office with nine or ten friends, but you may choose to have your partner (or another close friend or family member) get to know your midwives early in your care, or even at the initial meeting between you and your midwife. Other supporters might have the opportunity to get to know midwives or other midwifery clients at prenatal classes. If your midwives make some home visits, use those times to introduce your closest friends or family to them.

## What if You Can't Bring Them Around?

Despite your best efforts, some people may remain convinced that choosing a midwife to care for you, rather than opting for a doctor, means choosing inferior care. How you respond to this opposition has much to do with how you feel about yourself and your own choices. If you really think the midwifery option is for you, does the doubt of those around you undermine your own resolve, or does it make you feel uneasy about your relationship with those opposed? When Sarah experienced opposition from those close to her about her decision to have a homebirth, she recognized that their reaction stemmed from fear and concern. Even though she had no doubts about her choice, she still felt undermined by the opposition. She was just too close to the birth itself to try to explain why she felt homebirth was a safe option for her. It was especially difficult when some people suggested she had made choices based on her political beliefs rather than her child's health. In the end, it didn't matter what she said, she knew she would never be able to overcome the opposition and went about making her homebirth plans more privately.

Only you can decide whose opinion matters enough that it will truly influence your choices. Consider how much you are going to need these people's help in your pregnancy and your child's life, and whether their complete agreement with all your choices is possible or important.

### Jessica gains confidence in her choice

When I was thinking about having a midwife, I bounced the idea off a few friends. It was the wrong thing to do because they told me having a midwife was not necessary. Now I just tell people that a doctor is not necessary. Pregnancy is not an illness. You need support and guidance. That's what I think women need.

—*Jessica, mother of two*

But also remember that you and the baby's other parent will be the main people in your child's life. Your family, friends and neighbours play a supporting role—supporting you as the mother. However, you, and your partner, if you have one, are responsible for making decisions for your child—in the way you believe best, not in the way your sister or father-in-law or neighbour feels is best.

While it can be very difficult to parent in a way that is not endorsed by your regular cheering squad, it is more difficult to ignore your own feelings and beliefs about what is right for you and your baby. If this is your first child or you are seeking midwifery care because you want a different option, this may be good practice for other adversarial opinions you may encounter.

If you feel alone in your choice for midwifery care, speak to your midwives. In addition to helping you find ways to talk to your family and friends, they will probably be able to help you connect with other women or families who've made similar choices and possibly encountered similar opposition. Many women say that the other parents they've met while they were pregnant, or dealing with infants, remain among their best and closest friends. While it is extremely difficult to go through pregnancy, birth and the early days of parenthood without personal support, there is nothing that dictates that support come from your nearest and dearest.

## ◎ If You Want to Read More . . .

*Midwifery Is Catching*, by Eleanor Barrington (Toronto: NC Press Limited, 1985).

*The Mother of All Pregnancy Books: An All-Canadian Guide to Conception, Birth & Everything in Between*, by Ann Douglas (Toronto: CDG Books, 2000).

*Pregnancy and Birth: The Best Evidence*, by Joyce Barrett and Teresa Pitman (Toronto: Key Porter Books, 1999).

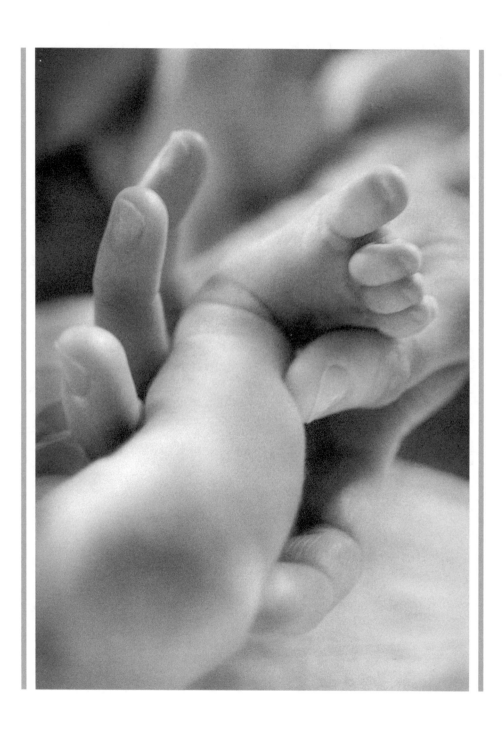

## Four

## The Midwife–Client Relationship

Whether you feel that nine months is an awfully long time to wait to see your baby, or that it just isn't enough time to prepare for such an awesome event, starting your prenatal care seems to propel you closer to the reality.

### When Do I Look for a Midwife?

Your chances of getting midwifery care will be best if you call the moment the second line appears on your pregnancy test. In most areas, midwives are in great demand. In unlegislated provinces, there may be only one or two midwives practising, or none at all. In legislated provinces—and particularly in provinces where the government not only recognizes midwifery but pays for it, too—even the larger number of midwives often cannot accommodate all the potential clients. Many practices have huge files of women they've turned away. One midwife said this situation almost requires that women roll out of bed the day they think they've conceived and make a phone call.

Some practices try to accommodate women who arrive later in pregnancy by leaving a fixed number of spots open on their roster of monthly births. Also, those big files containing the names of women that practices have to turn away are kept handy so that if a spot becomes available, they know who is next on the waiting list. On occasion, midwives are also able to accommodate women who decide late in pregnancy that they would pre-fer midwifery care.

If you're still undecided about the idea of midwifery, call anyway. Meet-ing a midwife face-to-face in her work environment, and having the oppor-tunity to ask all those questions, will probably give you the answers you need. You won't be wasting the midwife's time, because midwives book an extra-long introductory appointment to help you determine if their services are for you. In light of the high demand for midwives, it's worth investigat-ing early.

## Where Do I Look for a Midwife?

If you live in a province where midwifery is legislated (see Chapter 2) or in an urban centre, you can probably flip open the phone book and find a list-ing for a midwifery practice in your area or a professional body of mid-wives, such as a provincial association or a college of midwives.

If you live in a large city, you may call a midwifery practice only to dis-cover you aren't in its "catchment area"—that is, the geographic district it serves. Someone in the office will likely be able to tell you how to find the midwives who provide care in your neighbourhood.

In provinces where midwifery is legislated, many family doctors inform their pregnant patients about midwifery care and may refer them to a specific practice. Hospitals can also tell you which midwives have privi-leges on their maternity floors.

The Internet is a great place to get information about midwives who practise near you. Canadian midwifery organizations have a strong Web presence. The Canadian Association of Midwives has a listing of midwifery practices by province and territory, which can be accessed through their Web site. Some provincial and territorial associations of midwives have list-ings by area, too. Active consumer groups may have a Web site that will link to a local practice. The Web site for this book <www.midwiferyoption.ca> also links to many midwifery sites. These sites are also listed in the Appen-dix at the back of this book.

Many women come to midwifery because they know it will match their personal philosophies. Others hear about midwifery from family and friends who had their babies with midwives. The Maison de Naissance (birth centre) in Gatineau, Quebec, advertises midwifery on busboards. In Winnipeg, nurses at the local community health centres explain the midwifery and medical options to every woman who has a positive pregnancy test. An Ottawa midwife told us that a woman arrived at their office door, having walked into the medical clinic downstairs only to be told they didn't handle pregnancies. She knew nothing about midwifery care but wound up enthusiastically choosing a homebirth.

## When Does Midwifery Care Begin?

In many places it is standard practice for physicians to book the first visit with pregnant patients after 12 weeks or near the end of the first trimester.

This delay isn't part of midwifery care. If you know you are pregnant and the midwives have a spot on their roster for you, you will probably have your first visit almost immediately. This takes into account lifestyle and nutrition changes that may be necessary early in the pregnancy. It also encompasses the part of the pregnancy when many women experience nausea, mood swings and loss of energy. It means, as well, that midwives are there for the 10 to 20 percent of women who miscarry within their first 12 weeks. (See Chapter 5—Midwives and Pregnancy Loss.)

## The First Meeting

Some practices offer group information sessions to inform prospective clients about their services. If you live in Quebec, you can go on a group tour of your nearest birth centre before deciding whether to book an appointment with the midwives. For many people, the first encounter they have with their midwifery practice will be a face-to-face meeting with the midwife or midwives in their office.

Definitely, one of the most notable factors in your early care will be the opportunity to talk to your midwife without feeling rushed. Most midwives devote a particularly long time to their first getting-to-know-you meeting. Estimates from across the country range from 30 minutes to 75 minutes.

Your first visit will probably take place at your midwives' practice office. Many women note right away that the midwives' office usually has a welcoming atmosphere that is not at all clinical. There are usually beds, couches or upholstered benches instead of examining tables, and walls decorated with pictures of babies. You do not have to change into a gown or even take off any of your clothes during most of your visits.

At the first visit, much information is exchanged. The midwives will want to know practical details, such as when your baby is due, but they may also ask why you decided to consider midwifery care and what your hopes are for your pregnancy and birth. You will want to tell them about yourself and your hopes for this baby, as well as how their participation will provide the care that suits you and your family.

The midwife who meets you will explain the philosophy of midwifery care and how it is realized in her particular practice. You will probably hear the phrase "scope of practice," which describes what midwives can and cannot do in relation to elements of prenatal care, handling complications in labour and birth, choice of birth place, and so on.

If your provincial or territorial government does not fund midwifery, you will discuss payment options: how much you might pay for the services, what options might make midwifery more affordable for you, and when payments would be due.

The midwife you meet will explain the practice's approach to scheduling around birth and care. She will mention how many midwives could be involved in your care and who might assist in your birth, if you decide to work with the midwives.

On the first visit, you will probably feel you have a lot of information to process. For this reason, many midwifery practices have a policy of keeping the first visit open-ended so that you aren't forced to make a decision on the spot. At this first meeting, they may not go into any of the practical care elements or start a chart for you. Rather, they may wait until you feel sure that midwifery care is for you. If you are asked to take time to consider your answer, you will be told when the midwives will need your answer in order to ensure you a place in their care.

Some practices provide potential clients with a checklist of the midwives' philosophies. This is one way to make sure that women and their partners understand the concept of informed choice and that they agree to take responsibility for making informed decisions.

## Midwife Teams

Though you will probably be anxious to get to know the person who will be there when your baby is born, you will probably find yourself building relationships with more than one person at the midwifery office. Safe practice demands that two caregivers assist you and your baby at the moment of birth. In many places and situations, both attendants will be midwives, but some practices work with "second attendants"—a person who is trained to assist midwives in birthing. In a hospital birth in British Columbia, the second attendant might be a nurse from the Labour and Delivery floor.

Some midwives work in solo practices to provide prenatal and postpartum care, collaborating only at births, when they call on their second attendants for backup. The majority of midwives work in teams of two to four people that provide care to a client and ensure that she has access to support and assistance 24 hours a day, seven days a week throughout her care. Some practices assign a first midwife to each client. This midwife sees you most frequently, with another midwife acting as backup for some appointments and for the birth itself. Other practices share the care of each client among three or four midwives so that you get to know each midwife equally well. Two of the midwives will then attend your birth.

The midwife you meet on your first visit will explain the way that particular practice handles staffing and its way of helping you build a relationship with the individual midwives as your care progresses.

## Student Midwives

In provinces with educational programs, many midwifery practices supervise the practical education of student midwives. Depending on how far along they are in their studies, student midwives may be observers or participants in the care offered by these practices. A midwifery student in the final part of her training may also be referred to as a "clerk."

Miranda had reservations when she first heard that a student would be involved in her care. She imagined herself being asked the same questions again and again by a huge cast of characters and generally being treated like somebody's science project. The reality was vastly different. Midwifery students embrace the philosophies exemplified by the practising midwives and bring a great deal of enthusiasm, as well as individual talent, to their practical studies. Many women have told us that far from being an impediment to care, students were a beneficial addition to their midwifery experience.

## Developing a Relationship

For roughly 10 months you will visit with your midwives, share personal information of a physical and sometimes emotional nature, and be supported through your labour and child's birth and the first days of parenting. You are inviting your midwife into some of your most intimate moments. It is not surprising that some women feel very strongly about their relationship with their midwife.

Your trust and comfort in your midwife are certainly very important, as is her understanding of you, what you are hoping to achieve, and the way you approach things. A labour in which the mother has confidence in her abilities and feels unafraid and supported is less likely to be riddled with interventions. The midwives' presence is important not only because of their excellent clinical skills, but also because they know your pregnancy and can anticipate warning signs of problems and because they know your approach to decision-making. Similarly, after your baby is born, they know what your pregnancy and labour were like, they know what you had hoped for in your early days with your child, they know how you feel about yourself, and this helps them understand how you might handle the challenges a new baby inevitably presents.

Women seeking midwifery care come to it with different expectations regarding their relationship with their midwife. Women who express a desire to bond with someone whom they see as having shared experiences may be disturbed if they don't immediately feel some sort of "connection" or if their midwife doesn't seem to have the qualities they cherish in family or friends. Others feel concerned they will be asked to open up too soon to this new health care practitioner who is still a stranger. Some women don't feel they need a personal connection with a caregiver and come to midwives because they value their skills and the choices they provide.

It's important to remember that your midwife is there to support you and your personal circle and to help you and your baby get what you need during pregnancy, birth and in the postpartum period. She needs to *be there for you*, not *be you*. A good midwife should be able to support you fully, no matter what her own background. A midwife once told Sarah she thought an excellent midwife was one who could reflect her client's own beliefs and values.

### Understanding the midwife's role

When I found out that someone I knew in high school was going to be one of my midwives, I thought I might feel a little strange. I thought I wouldn't want to be so exposed in front of her, because I knew her during all those silly teenage years. Then the whole friendship thing vanished. I didn't even remember I knew her in high school. The midwife relationship was so much stronger. She was my midwife, and that was it. She was looking at my hemorrhoids! To come away from that experience not feeling humiliated was amazing. If you flash me back 15 years, I would never have believed it.

A midwife is so different to me than a friend. You don't have to worry about the egos and each other's feelings. With girlfriends, you're treading on thinner ground. With midwives, it's just for you. There is a friendship and a relationship, but it's different.

—Jessica, mother of two

What if, after a visit or two, you find it difficult to imagine revealing yourself physically or emotionally to this person? Does this mean she is the wrong midwife for you?

Probably not. The trust and comfort that women describe feeling with their midwives results from many meetings and conversations over the course of about 10 months. It's the result of the good work midwives do, the skills you come to recognize as your pregnancy progresses, combined with the attention they give at your appointments and at any other time you need their expertise. You will not feel your midwife knows you on your first or second visit, because she doesn't. What you should feel is that she is willing to try.

**A quiet place to consider the pregnancy**

It seems I spend my life rushing: juggling children's lessons, appointments, work obligations, household responsibilities and social engagements. Yet when I am at the midwife's, I never feel rushed. The atmosphere is homey, the people friendly, the pace relaxed. Her clinic is a sanctuary to me, full of expectation. I look forward to being there.

—Rebecca, mother of three

Aside from time, talk is the other crucial element to building a relationship with your midwife. Midwives' appointments usually last much longer than doctors' appointments, and the conversations tend to be far-ranging. One of the first things many women mention when speaking about their midwives is how wonderful it was to be asked, "How are you doing?" It's not a standard question in the medical approach to prenatal care. Instead of merely finding out what is going on with you physically, the midwives want to know how you are feeling as your baby grows and the birth approaches. They recognize that birth is a life event that involves many elements besides how big your belly is. If your partner just lost his job and you are wondering how you will pay for this baby, if you've just been offered the promotion of your dreams but it requires you go back to work in three months, if your father has just died, all these things will be affecting you. Talk about them if you want to and if you can.

### Feeling comfortable at the midwives' office

We alternated appointments with our two midwives so that we could get to know both of them equally well. I'll never forget both of their offices. They had each converted part of their home into an office space. The spaces felt like someone's living room. You entered through a wooden front door (or back door), not some glass and chrome safety door at the local clinic. This is all very important. I dislike doctors' offices and their bad art, ugly paint jobs, long waiting times and silly magazine racks. I generalize, I know. I'm sure there is some midwife out there who has an ugly office, but I have yet to see it.

I feel like the restaurant critic who only talks about the decor and what the service was like. However, it underpins the major difference between the experience with a doctor's care for our first child and our birth experience with midwives.

The really great thing is that the appointments were an hour long, which only reinforced the need for comfortable surroundings. This gave us plenty of time to go over our questions, and I really got to enjoy our visits with our midwives.

—Chris, father of two

Similarly, midwives are not so pressed for time that they can't laugh with you. For most of us, having a baby is something to be celebrated. Getting to know your sense of humour is good for your caregivers, because many times during pregnancy and the first few days with a baby, you need to be encouraged to laugh!

As your pregnancy proceeds and your midwives get to know you better, you should begin to feel that you have that connection you had hoped for.

**Unexpected support**

My first meeting with my midwife was a bit disconcerting. I found her a bit cold. I decided to go ahead with it anyway, since overall I felt I trusted her. She seemed very knowledgeable and intelligent, if not that warm. When I think back to that impression of coldness, I'm amazed, since during a really difficult birth and postpartum period, my midwife turned out to be the person who kept me sane. She offered a lot of great advice and many hugs.

*—Pam, mother of one, born by C-section*

## When the Fit Isn't Right

Our experiences with our midwives have been resoundingly good, as have the vast majority of experiences of our friends, acquaintances and the women we have met across the country in the course of writing this book. That said, there are times when the midwife–client relationship does not go smoothly.

You want to meet the challenge of labour and birth feeling good about your care. If you do not feel confident about your midwives and comfortable with them, their presence will become a hindrance rather than a help. That kind of relationship negates everything midwifery stands for.

So what to do? First, consider why you feel uncomfortable. Are you concerned about a lack of responsiveness and attentiveness in your caregiver, or are you troubled by care that seems clinically inadequate? Would you prefer and feel more comfortable with medical care? Are you considering your midwife's competence as a health professional or are you asking for her to be something more? If, after considering the reasons for your discomfort, you still feel that midwifery care is for you, you will need to find ways to address your concerns.

The first step is to discuss them with the midwife in question. This is often easier said than done, particularly if you feel the problem with the midwife is a lack of communication. It may help to write down your feelings or to bring another person with you for the conversation. If you still feel unable to discuss your concerns, it may be possible to address them with another midwife in your care group. She might be able to make suggestions about how to approach your midwife.

This does not have to be a horrible experience. Like all of us, midwives need feedback to grow, and learning when things aren't working is part of that. Some clients happily report that a conversation about what isn't working changes everything and brings the midwife and mother closer to their communication goals. If this does not work, then your midwife will encourage you to consider finding another caregiver: a midwife, if appropriate, or a physician.

If talk isn't enough to save the experience, then you should see if another midwife is available at the practice. Perhaps someone with whom you feel more comfortable can take on the majority of your care.

## When Do I Page?

Your team of midwives provides care 24 hours a day, seven days a week. Most midwives can be reached via their pager, though some prefer to give out their home or mobile phone numbers instead.

Some women hold on to those numbers for their entire period of care and only call the midwives when they know they are in labour. But other midwifery clients will need to page their midwives on occasion throughout their pregnancy and during the first few days with their baby, when they encounter situations that require urgent assistance outside office hours.

Of course, you do not want to bother your midwives with inappropriate interruptions. Many questions and concerns can be brought to your next visit or wait until office hours—3:00 A.M. is not the time to call about your hemorrhoids. However, it is important to call in an urgent situation. The midwives will give you an indication of situations in which you should page them. For example, if you start to bleed, if there is a sudden absence of fetal movement or a leak of fluids, call them. But other unpredictable situations also occur. If you are concerned enough to consider a trip to a walk-in clinic or emergency ward, you should first contact your midwives. They will help you determine whether this trip is necessary. If a trip to the hospital is necessary, one of your midwives may be able to meet you there.

## Missed Appointments

Many midwives have dual work lives. They have visits scheduled during the day and often stay up all night while one of their clients has her baby. For this reason, they will probably have to reschedule an appointment from time to time, or another midwife involved in your care may meet you instead. Many midwives recommend you contact them before you head out to your visit, just to make sure they are not at a birth or recovering from one that occurred the night before. However, some midwives arrange the practice schedule so that the midwife who is not on-call for births does prenatal appointments.

## Doctor Consultations and Shared Doctor–Midwife Care

Most women who begin to see certain midwives will remain solely in their care throughout pregnancy, birth and the postpartum period. However, if a woman develops complications during her pregnancy that require the attention of a physician, the midwives will consult with a doctor about the best course of action for their client. If you wind up needing to see a doctor at some point, it doesn't necessarily mean your midwifery care will come to an end. Although a doctor will sometimes assume all further care, this is not a foregone conclusion. A consultation with a doctor may be a one-time occurrence, or there may be periodic visits while the doctor makes sure that no further intervention is required. Sometimes doctors and midwives can arrange to share a woman's care. They may arrange parallel appointments or have midwives attend the meetings with the doctor. Sometimes, depending on how advanced your pregnancy is, your midwife can stay on as labour support and reassume your care postpartum.

## Combined Doctor–Midwife Care

In provinces and territories without midwifery legislation, midwives must practise in a home setting. They cannot provide women with access to blood tests, fetal diagnostic tests (such as ultrasounds or amniocentesis), or prescribe basic pregnancy-related drugs, nor can they guarantee a smooth entry into hospital should it be required during labour. If this is the situation in your area, you may want to visit your doctor periodically as your pregnancy progresses so that you can access some of the mainstream medical options and have a referring physician on your charts in case you do need to go to hospital during labour. Your family doctor may be the appropriate person to provide this care, but if he or she disapproves of your decision to have midwives or to give birth at home, then your midwife may be able to suggest a doctor who will be more supportive of your choices. For example, in Nova Scotia, where midwifery is not legislated, sometimes it is possible to work quite closely with doctors. Midwives may be able to provide charted information to the doctor so that women do not have to have double appointments.

## Prenatal Classes

As your pregnancy progresses, your conversations with your midwives—either one-on-one, or with your partner in attendance—will give you a good indication of what to expect during labour and birth. This may feel like sufficient preparation.

However, many women still like to enrol in a prenatal class. In your visits you may cover much of the class curriculum, but these classes offer the benefits of camaraderie as well as information. Even if your partner has been able to attend all of your visits with the midwives, it can be really reassuring to talk to other families who are also waiting anxiously for the beginning of labour.

**Prenatal class benefits**

Physically, I could have given birth with no classes at all, but the classes helped me to wrap my mind around what was going to happen and helped us talk about it together in specific and concrete ways.

*—Susan, mother of three*

Some midwives offer their own classes for clients; those who don't can often suggest classes that will suit families who have opted for a midwife-assisted birth. If your midwife doesn't know of any classes in your area, try to discover which instructors are familiar with midwifery clients. If you are planning a homebirth and your classmates and teacher are focused on how quickly to call for the epidural, the class is likely to frustrate you rather than prepare you for a confident birth experience. If you hear things in class that seem at odds with what your midwives have told you, be sure to bring this up with your midwives at the next appointment.

Many prenatal classes focus on the physical preparation for labour and birth. Others explore birth from a spiritual perspective, concentrating on the environment and ritual you may want to create for your child's birth. Some classes focus on the pregnancy, downplaying the postpartum period, and others take a more holistic approach.

Class content can be determined by the instructor, by the organization giving the classes or by a particular method of childbirth, such as the Lamaze or Bradley approaches. The Lamaze approach to birth involves using imagery and meditation to help you get beyond the pain of labour. The Bradley Method focuses on coaching techniques used by the woman's partner (it is also called Husband-Coached Childbirth) and encourages the woman to concentrate on what is going on in her body. Both approaches are based on the idea that birth is a natural process that should be free of interventions. While these methods have many benefits, remember that in midwifery care, your caregivers' approach is tailored to your choices and needs rather than adhering to a formula. During labour, your midwives will be guided by whatever particular techniques work for you at the time.

## Home Visit(s)

Home visits are one of the great bonuses of midwifery care. Even if you do not plan to have a homebirth, most midwives will arrange for at least one of your prenatal visits to take place at your home. This usually happens later in the pregnancy, around 36 weeks, though some midwives prefer to conduct their visits at the clients' homes on a regular basis.

This type of visit allows the midwives to get to know the way to your home so that they are ready for the "I think I'm in labour" call, when they will probably come to check you. And, of course, the midwives will be visiting you at home after your baby arrives.

Most women love the home visit(s). It lets you welcome the midwives into your space and allows them to get to know you better. You can take this opportunity to introduce your personal support people, if they haven't already accompanied you on a visit to the midwives' office. If you plan to have your children attend the birth, this is a good time for them to meet the midwives. A home visit can also help families planning a homebirth imagine labour in a more detailed way.

### ◎ *If You Want to Read More . . .*

*Birthing From Within: An Extra-Ordinary Guide to Childbirth Preparation*, by Pam England and Rob Horowitz (Albuquerque, New Mexico: Partera Press, 1998).

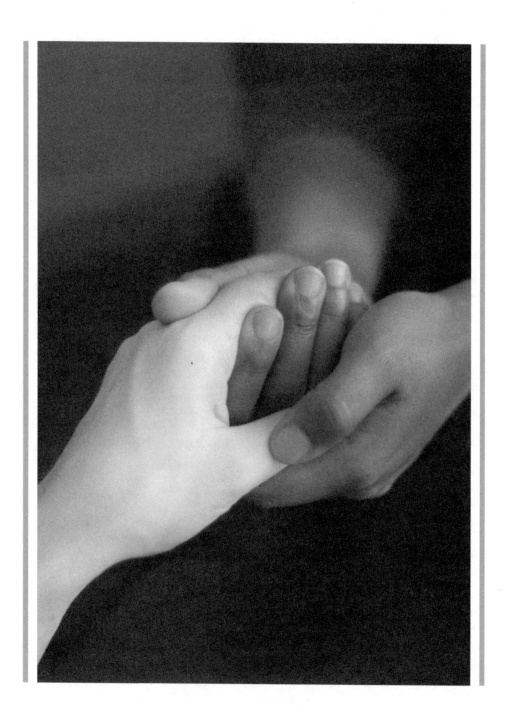

## Five

### Midwives and Pregnancy Loss

Sometimes losing babies is a part of pregnancy, and dealing with pregnancy loss, particularly miscarriages, is an important part of a midwife's job.

**Support during an early miscarriage**

When I became pregnant the first time, I immediately contacted a midwife—a woman I found through the phone book. But before my first appointment, I miscarried. The midwife offered sympathy and support and said I could use her library if I wanted to read about miscarriage, grief or conception. When I became pregnant again two months later, I called her again, this time with some apprehension about pregnancy.

—*Susan, mother of three*

As noted previously, obstetricians often don't see women until they are 12 weeks pregnant, by which time they are less likely to suffer a miscarriage. If you are in the care of a midwife and you suspect you are miscarrying, you have someone to call for care, advice and some comfort. She may be able to arrange any necessary tests, and will talk you through the experience of waiting for the results. When Sarah started to bleed at 11 weeks, she called her midwife, who was able to provide her with the information she needed to decide whether to stay at home or go to the hospital for tests and treatment. This support and clinical care helped Sarah immeasurably through an extremely difficult time.

### How midwives help through difficult times

One of my miscarriages was at 22 weeks in a hospital in Montreal. I had no family around to support me. I wish it could have been possible at least to have a midwife at the hospital even if it was a *quallanat* (non-Inuit) midwife. I had another miscarriage in Puvirnituq. It was somewhat easier than in Montreal because I was not alone. I had support from the Inuit midwives. But it was still too far from my home. I would have preferred to stay in Inukjuak.

I think midwives do a lot, even in the south. They listen to the woman and try to understand.

—*Brenda, mother of one*

One thing that some women who have miscarried lament is that their loss is difficult to discuss with people, because some will say the baby was never "real." Yet the woman who has lost her developing child can feel devastated. Midwives understand that having a miscarriage is a traumatic experience, even if it happens to many women. The midwives' recognition that your experience of pregnancy is just as valid as that of someone who carried her baby to full-term can help immeasurably in dealing with miscarriage and deciding whether or when to try again.

### Talking about loss

In my second pregnancy (my first with midwives) I went for an ultrasound appointment at 21 weeks. The ultrasound technician left the room and came back crying, saying, "I've called your midwife. She's going to meet you here." Then she walked away. So we walked around the hospital, pretty much knowing that something had happened. Our midwife joined us. She shared our sadness and confirmed that our baby was dead. She then found us an obstetrician who had chosen to have midwifery care for her own baby. This doctor opened her office early three days in a row to soften my cervix so that we could get prepared for an induction. Later I was induced at the hospital, and when the baby was actually born, our midwife caught the baby because the obstetrician was attending another woman.

My midwife called me for the next few weeks to see how I was doing and how my husband, James, was dealing with the situation. I needed that contact because of the connection she had to our lives. She knew everything that had happened to us, so I could talk to her without having to explain anything. It changed the way that experience shaped our lives. It made it part of life, instead of a devastating experience we couldn't talk about.

A few months later I was able to visit her to give her a Christmas present and tell her that I was pregnant again.

*—Mandy, mother of five*

Midwives can also be there to support women who have the terrible experience of losing their babies after the job of labour and birth is done. As health care professionals who work within a larger community, midwives can help you gain access to additional services you may need for ongoing care. Midwives know the history of their client's pregnancy and birth, but they also know that woman as a person. This connection may help the woman and her family to better understand and accept the loss they have suffered.

### Losing a baby after birth

Sean arrived five days early. We had just moved to our house, and my mom had just arrived from Israel. We were unpacking boxes the whole day, and later that night I started having contractions. I called my midwife, but the contractions were still far apart. So she told me we could just hang out and wait. When things got more intense, our midwives came and checked me. I had dilated just one centimetre! We all tried to get some sleep. Then I suddenly woke up again with a horrible pain and started screaming. After that, things started to move more quickly; within two hours I had dilated to eight centimetres. I went into the birth pool with my partner, Ryan. I leaned against him through a short transition, then I pushed for about 20 minutes. Then Sean was born in the pool. I found breastfeeding to be difficult. Sean was very sleepy and couldn't nurse for more than a minute or two. By the third day, the problem seemed worse and the midwives decided to come early for their daily visit.

When they checked the baby, my primary midwife said he was too cool. They wrapped him, called the hospital, and said that we needed to go right away to see the pediatrician. On the way, Sean became quieter and quieter in the car. When we got there, the student midwife took him in the elevator, and as soon as the doors opened, she ran down the hall. The nurses and doctors pushed us out of the room and they put him into an incubator.

We were so confused, and I still didn't feel too worried. I was in a different land. Three midwives were sitting with us, then this doctor came to see us. I will never forget his voice. He said, "Your child is very, very sick." I thought, No, it happens only in the movies. I couldn't accept that it could happen to us.

The doctor explained that one half of Sean's heart had never developed. It couldn't be seen on the routine ultrasound that we had at 18 weeks. He told us we were going to have to make a decision. While the baby was in the womb, he was fine. But in the days after his birth, his heart couldn't function and get enough oxygen to his lungs and to his blood. He was so fatigued he could barely nurse or breathe. They could try a series of surgeries, but even if they worked, he would have brain damage that might be severe.

At first, we didn't think, we just wanted them to do everything they could to save him. But the midwives walked us through all our options. I thought to myself about how much I loved him, and who would I be keeping him alive for? Would it be for his sake or for me, because I couldn't let go of him? When I realized that if I loved him I had to let him go, I was able to make the decision. It wasn't easy, because he wouldn't be with me. But I knew what I had to do.

We had to decide when we wanted to do it and how we wanted to do it. We had him transferred to the children's hospital. He was all connected to tubes everywhere, intravenous drips and morphine. We went home and had a sleep. Then we went back to the hospital. We read to him and we played music. I held his hand, because, when I had been being stitched up after the birth, it was quite painful, but one of the midwives had given me her hand, and it had relaxed me so much. I had never realized how much comfort can come from that simple physical contact with someone. So I held Sean's hand while he lay in the incubator. My mom and I told him about his family in Israel. And each of the midwives spoke to him.

The midwives stayed with us all that day. We cried together, and they sat quietly in the corner of the room. They did not interfere; they just took pictures for us, brought us water and looked after everything. In the afternoon, the nurse asked if we were ready to disconnect, and so we held him and said goodbye.

You know, I feel that without them I would never have come through it. I would still have been frustrated and angry that my baby had died. We fell, and these hands lifted us up, just before we hit the ground.

The midwives came to our house the next morning, and one of them came, every day, for a month. They listened to us, and they helped us talk about all the good things about him. They never stated an opinion; they just sat there and nodded while we talked. Later, the midwives said, "Let us know if you'd like us to come tomorrow." Then they came once a week; then once a month. Eventually our need to see them all the time faded away.

I had my daughter Maya two years later, and I can talk about her birth with a smile. The midwives helped me work through all my worries. She was born in a birthing pool in the same room that Sean had been born in. The birth was so much easier, and I was so much happier after she was born. The midwives were there for that too, for the part of me that is like any other mother with a new baby.

—*Merav, mother of two*

## ◈ *If You Want to Read More . . .*

*Trying Again: A Guide to Pregnancy After Miscarriage, Stillbirth and Infant Loss*, by Ann
Douglas (Toronto: Taylor Publishing, 2000).

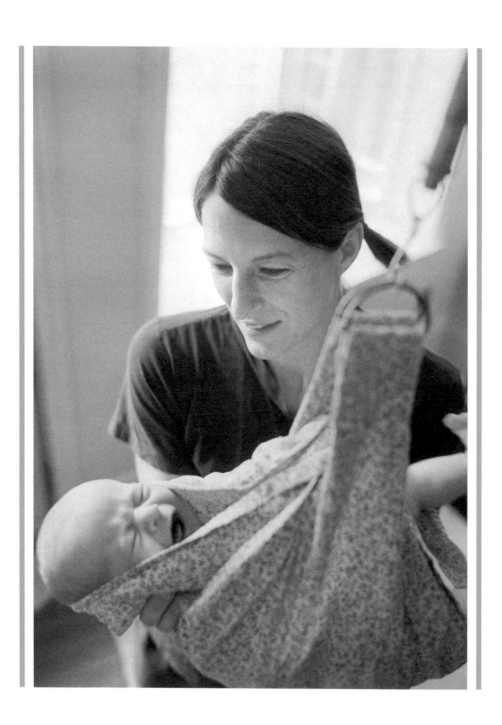

## Six

### Your Care with Midwives

On the first visit following your decision to have midwifery care, the midwives will record your pregnancy history—past pregnancies, births and so on—and any particular physical concerns you have. They will probably also note your weight and blood pressure to establish a baseline for future changes as your pregnancy progresses. They will begin a chart that will record your progress from visit to visit. In provinces where midwifery is legislated, some of the information in your chart will be submitted to the Ministry of Health. In provinces that do not have legislation, some of your prenatal records will be shared with your doctor to keep him or her informed of your progress.

#### Regular Visits

After the initial get-to-know-you visit, most midwives book between a half hour and an hour for regular visits with clients. Your visits will probably take place once a month for the first two trimesters, then every other week until week 36, and then once a week during the last month of your pregnancy. This basic pattern is set and followed by the medical establishment and most midwives. However, some midwives adjust this pattern to suit the needs and preferences of their clients. For example, during the first two trimesters, midwives at one practice in Quebec meet clients every five weeks instead of every four so that they can provide extra visits during the postpartum period. Some meet every five weeks, then every three weeks, and then every week.

At your appointments, the midwives will guide you through a discussion of your overall health and how it is evolving over the course of your pregnancy. There is no doubt that following a healthy lifestyle will help your baby, but staying healthy is important for you, too. Your body will go through rapid changes, and taking care of it will help you in the pregnancy and birth as well as the postpartum period.

Regular checkups are useful for detecting any problems that may develop. These may range from discomforts to serious conditions. We cannot possibly mention them all here, but we have touched on some of the most common ones.

Early on, you will probably discuss whether you and your baby will get adequate nutrition from your current diet or whether your eating habits need to be altered. Do you need supplements or is your current meal plan adequate? Have you built enough exercise into your day? Very active women may want to discuss whether their current form of exercise should be maintained or adjusted as their pregnancy progresses. Your midwives will monitor your blood pressure at each appointment. They will also keep track of any fluctuations in regular tests, such as regular urine tests, occasional blood tests and weigh-ins, if you have them. They will discuss the rest that you need and how you might get it.

Midwives note your progress from appointment to appointment in detailed records, in the same way as a family doctor or obstetrician. However, longer appointments and a commitment to choice throughout your care means that midwives might seem less prescriptive when it comes to advice. In midwifery care, you are unlikely to get a lecture about gaining more weight than the published guidelines recommend, nor will you receive a set list of what to eat at each meal. Instead, midwives take an approach to your care that factors in your previous patterns and experience.

If your lifestyle includes some more pronounced risk factors for your pregnancy, such as alcohol consumption, smoking or drug use, your midwives will help you develop a plan to improve the potential outcome for you and your baby.

Longer appointments and an approach tailored to the individual foster an environment where mother-to-be and midwives can discuss intimate topics. These might include sexuality during pregnancy or how the pregnancy is affecting relationships (with partners, family and friends) and self-esteem. Some women feel comfortable addressing these topics and find that their midwives really help them come to terms with what the pregnancy and impending birth mean to them. Other women prefer to approach their appointments in a more diagnostic way. The midwives are open to both these preferences and are committed to serving their clients in the way that is best for the women themselves.

**More to know than you thought . . .**

For my second and third kids I remember thinking, I don't need all these midwifery appointments. What are we going to talk about in that hour? I have nothing to talk about. Everything is fine.

Then I would get to the appointment and it would take the hour. We would talk and I would think, It is a good thing we talked about that because I found out this and that. I felt reassured about things I hadn't yet realized I was worried about.

—*Janet, mother of three*

Many women note with surprise and relief that their midwives do not stand over them as they weigh themselves or hand over a plastic bottle for a urine sample. There is an indignity in being asked to pee in a cup and place it on a shelf. The fewer times one has to do this the better. So the midwives may offer you the opportunity to test yourself.

Most clients can note the numbers on a scale and differentiate between the colours on a test strip that measures traces of protein, blood and sugar in the urine. Many women prefer this opportunity to test themselves, report the results and consult with the midwives if results appear unusual. In some ways this highlights a fundamental difference between midwifery care and traditional medical care.

In later pregnancy, midwifery clients may also administer their own vaginal swabs in private. Midwives will carefully describe the best way to do this.

In parts of the country with midwifery legislation, routine midwifery care also includes blood tests that can identify or confirm your blood type, iron levels and glucose. Such tests can also detect hepatitis B, syphilis or immunity to rubella.

Midwives will explain tests that may occur during your care. You should know what the test is for, how it is done and what the results might mean. It's important that the midwives talk to you about each procedure, not just to answer questions you may have but also to provide vital information that may inspire questions about the progress of your pregnancy and your care.

## Choices

Choice is being pitched to us for everything from cable packages to burger toppings, so it's easy to be cynical about the idea. But if you are already a parent, you know that making choices for your children is an all-consuming job. If you are a first-time parent, you're about to find that out.

Throughout your care, your midwives will provide you with information about various choices you need to make. Some of them will be fairly major and straightforward choices, such as whether to have your baby at home or in hospital. Others are smaller and may come as a surprise. Maybe you knew that most people have an ultrasound in their second trimester. Now you have to decide if *you* want one. Thinking about this may raise lots of questions. Why would you want one? What are the benefits to the baby, to you, to your partner? Why might you *not* want one? What are the potential drawbacks of such a test? Why might you want to buck convention and forgo the procedure?

This is the time when many women turn to their midwives and say, "I don't know. What did *you* do?" Your midwife may tell you. She may not. Your midwife made her choices based not only on her professional expertise but also on her personal preference: she made an informed choice that was right for her. That doesn't mean that her choice will be right for you. Most midwives are very aware that women could be inclined to follow the midwife's plan instead of determining their own. To help you make a decision that is difficult or contentious, your midwife will probably be able to recommend books on the subject and may possibly refer you to other mothers with a variety of experiences and responses to the situation you are debating. Sarah's midwife explained that it is hard for women to realize that often there is no "right decision," just one that is right for that woman, her experience and her body.

There are not always right or wrong answers, but there will probably be answers that are right or wrong for you. Most women embrace the concept of making the right choices for themselves, based on the best and most current information. It assumes that you are the person responsible for your body, your care and your baby. This just makes sense. But the reality of making choices is that some of them will be hard. Sometimes giving consent without thinking, for tests and practices that are "routine" or "standard," is easier—in the short run. Though the constant insistence on choice can sometimes be difficult, the confidence it will give you in your own decision-making ability will be something you appreciate when your child is born and when he or she starts needing you as a strong advocate, whether in the sandbox or in the principal's office.

### The challenge of informed choice

Not being rushed means having the time to get to know one another, to develop trust, and to have my questions answered. I always feel heard. This does, however, come at the price of added responsibility. Tests and procedures that were simply taken for granted in my doctor's care require decisions with the midwife. While I appreciate the information, and am amazed at not having heard much of it before, I occasionally find myself secretly wondering if the empowerment of informed choice is truly preferable to letting someone else make decisions for me. Why do I always have to be the grown-up? But deep down, I know it is.

—*Rebecca, mother of three*

## Choosing Your Place of Birth

Some midwives do not have options about where they provide care. In provinces without legislation, midwives are not integrated into the hospital system, and in Quebec, midwives may only attend births in specialized birth centres. But for many women, choosing midwifery means choosing where to have their babies.

Because midwives need to balance the demand for home and hospital births, you may be asked very early in your care—or even when you first call to inquire about care—where you intend to have your baby. It is important to know that your feelings in this matter can evolve over the course of your pregnancy. If your comfort level grows to permit the possibility of a home-birth, or if circumstances, or new feelings, demand that your planned homebirth be moved to the hospital, no one is going to insist that you stick to your initial preference. (For help with your home versus hospital decision, refer to Chapter 7.)

## Midwives and the Use of Tests and Technology

In areas with midwifery legislation, midwifery clients have access to the same tests and technologies as women in a doctor's care. During your pregnancy, midwives can order tests and prescribe some drugs for pregnancy-related conditions. So you might indeed find yourself choosing to have the same tests as your friend who has a doctor's care.

Many women see midwives' access to technology as a positive thing, but others find this phenomenon troubling and worry that the connection some Canadian midwives have to the medical system will adversely affect their care, interfering with a more "natural" approach.

What does access to the system mean to you and your baby?

Ultimately, it probably means more choice and more opportunity to decide what will work for you. If you want genetic testing for your baby, or you are Rh negative and require injections, you can access these services through your midwife. If your labour progresses in such a way that the use of technology will mean better outcomes for you or your baby, the midwives' ability to tap into the existing medical system will help the transition happen smoothly, with less disruption to the labouring mom.

One of the greatest fears women have about testing or the use of technology concerns the domino effect—one questionable intervention that then leads to the use of another and another. The midwives help you consider the possible outcomes of a test or technology. They can also help you identify your feelings about certain technological options before they present themselves so that you are not making hurried decisions in a moment of confusion or fear.

### As normal as possible

My midwives provided what no one else could. They helped us negotiate our way through a pregnancy that wasn't normal and helped make it as normal as possible—to allow it to be "un-normal" in the way that it needed to be, to attend to the particularities of the situation, and also to respect the ways in which things *could* still be normal.

I got pregnant when I was 35, so my partner and I had a long talk with the midwives about the options for genetic screening. Then we thought long and hard about what we wanted to do. We decided against all tests except for ultrasound. But we thought that would be our entire genetic screening.

When we went for our ultrasound at 18 weeks, the technician said, "I can't see the bladder filling." He called a doctor in, but the doctor couldn't see it either. They didn't tell us what it meant. They recommended we talk with our midwives and suggested that we schedule another ultrasound. Before we scheduled another test, we needed more information. We wanted to know why we needed another ultrasound and what the first results meant. The midwives called up people they knew to do some research for us; they also tried to find information about the first test results before we decided to do more.

The midwives told us that it could be something called "bladder exstrophy," which is a congenital abnormality that is surgically reparable but can have long-term physical and possible emotional effects. Also, there were some references in the reading we did that linked the condition to all sorts of things that could make for a really different quality of life for my baby.

The potential consequences were serious enough that my partner and I knew we would terminate the pregnancy if the condition were to seriously affect our child's quality of life. We also knew that even if we didn't choose to terminate, the condition might influence our birth plans. I had planned to have the baby at home, but if I were going to have a child with a physical anomaly, would it still be appropriate? Clearly the condition raised many questions. We decided to go ahead with the second ultrasound.

We had a great sonographer. He did an internal and external ultrasound, and said, "It's clear to me that your baby has bladder exstrophy," but that was really all the information he gave us. Had I not spoken to my midwives, if I hadn't had that information, I wouldn't have known what he meant. Having that information from the midwives made a huge difference to me.

I was 19 weeks pregnant: as you can imagine, the question on our minds was, are we going through with this pregnancy or not? All of a sudden, you've got a baby that has a major abnormality; you know something but not that much about it, and part of the difficultly is that it's on a continuum—you don't know if you will get a best-case scenario or a worst-case one.

I've always felt that a woman should have the right to abort a pregnancy if that is right for her. Until I was in that position, so late in pregnancy, I don't think I ever appreciated what a torment that choice could be. All of my person really wanted it to be O.K. to have the baby. Intellectually, I was prepared to do otherwise. If that was the right decision, I would make it. But in my heart, I didn't want to have to make it.

Based on our ultrasound, our pediatric surgeon was able to assure us that our baby did not have the most serious form of exstrophy. That made us realize we could handle this. We could make a decision based on our knowledge of the condition and what was best for us and for our child.

We were told the baby would require surgery within 72 hours of his birth, but that prenatal care could be normal. So one of the things the diagnosis did for us was to allow us to plan for his birth. We made plans that I would never have been able to make, had I not known so much ahead of time.

There were a number of things the baby would need after the birth. With this condition, the bladder is turned inside out. The tissue, therefore, is exposed in a way that's really vulnerable. The condition is very rare (about 1 in 30,000), so many people, even in the medical community, are not familiar with it or the most current treatments for it. As a result we went through a process of education with our midwives about it. The midwives arranged for us to meet and make plans with the other people who would be involved in our baby's care. For instance, they advised the obstetrician and pediatric staff to ensure that certain things were done and that others were not; really simple things: "Don't clamp the cord, use a tie on it, so you don't have that plastic on there that's going to scratch the bladder. Don't put anything on the bladder, use a vapour dome on it. There's no reason this mother can't be with her child afterwards. There's nothing that precludes her from taking the baby on her belly and nursing." We heard from other parents we contacted that precious first moments in their births were lost because people saw something they didn't understand. Our midwives played an incredible role in the birth, both in facilitating our learning experience and in educating themselves about bladder extrophy in order to help us have a good birth. They helped attend to our baby's particular needs without missing what was normal about his birth. Without our combined efforts, none of this would have been achieved.

The midwives were also really helpful in allowing our son to be with me after the birth. I really wanted to avoid a C-section, because that would have meant I would recover in one hospital while my baby went on to another. The midwives helped me have the baby without a C-section, even though it meant other interventions, like inducing labour so the baby would come when the doctors would be available. Within two or three hours of the birth he was moved to the pediatric hospital for the surgery.

So much of the groundwork for my son's birth was laid by the midwives. They told the other caregivers: "These are the concerns of our client. She is very well-informed about her child's condition, but she is also very concerned that we not forget her baby is normal in many ways." For me, that was very important because I had seen so many pictures of kids with bladder exstrophy that I couldn't imagine my child's face when I tried to picture him: all I could see was the bladder exstrophy. But it was important also to see that this was just a pregnancy. When he was born, everybody in the room just looked at him and said, "What a beautiful baby." Nobody gasped. Nobody said, "Oh, what a shame. What a sad thing." And then I said, "Oh, yes, and that's classic bladder exstrophy, just as we knew it would be." When he was born, I could truly rejoice.

*—Colette, mother of one*

It is also important to remember that the availability of tests and technology and their actual use are not the same thing. Making use of testing and technology is simply another possibility for the midwifery client.

## Standard Prenatal Testing

Pregnancy is mysterious, unavoidably so. Sure, your belly will expand, and during your pregnancy, you'll be able to see and feel flutters, kicks and rolls. Modern science allows many opportunities to peek at what's happening inside your uterus, but what we can interpret from these investigations is still relatively murky. Deciding whether or not to opt for prenatal tests, or which tests to select, can involve fact-finding and soul-searching. Whatever your initial feelings about prenatal testing, you will probably need time to consider all the possibilities and information in order to decide what is right for you.

While some tests are routinely suggested, others are available if you choose. For example, midwives will almost always recommend at least a blood test to rule out Rh negativity but will make ultrasound available as a choice. At every visit your midwife will measure your *fundus* (uterus), but the trip to the scale can be an option rather than a routine. Midwives' guiding philosophy dictates that they make you aware of your options, the current research and how the possibilities for testing might fit into your overall approach to growing and birthing your baby.

Here are some tests you will probably be introduced to early in your care. For most people, these tests will not seem too intrusive. If you have a concern about the necessity of any of these procedures, however, make sure you fully discuss it with your midwife.

### Weigh-ins

Some midwives will suggest regular weigh-ins. These help them to note the changes in your body as your pregnancy progresses. Though they may contribute to information about your overall health, weigh-ins are not necessary if they make you uncomfortable. Measurements of weight gained each month are sometimes used in mainstream pregnancy literature as a marker and may create a false sense of success or failure. These numbers are averages and do not take into account individual bodies. Midwives recognize that each woman is different.

### Fundal Measurement

The midwives will measure the growth of your uterus by stretching a cloth or paper tape measure from the top of your pelvis to the top of your uterus. By a fluke of nature, the pregnant belly grows about one centimetre per week over the course of a pregnancy, although this varies slightly from one woman to another. Unlike weight gain, this test actually measures the growth of your uterus and the baby inside. A variation from your own pattern might warrant further testing.

### Blood Tests

Early in pregnancy, blood tests are usually done to determine or verify your blood type. This is an important standard test. If you have a negative blood type and the baby's father has a positive type, your baby may also have a positive blood type. This may pose a problem if the baby's blood cells and yours intermingle, which can easily happen if there is a trauma during pregnancy, such as placental abruption, or during amniocentesis. The Rh negative mother will then produce antibodies to the baby's Rh positive blood cells, putting this baby and future ones at risk. This condition causes anemia in the baby, and anemia can lead to a range of problems from severe jaundice at birth, which could cause brain damage, to stillbirth.

The treatment is simple: give all Rh negative mothers an injection of anti-D gamma globulin during pregnancy and immediately after birth or a miscarriage. Depending on where you live, these injections may be administered by a midwife or a nurse.

A mother's blood is also routinely tested for glucose, hemoglobin (iron), hepatitis B, syphilis, and immunity to rubella. These tests provide indicators of many conditions that can be watched for and treated as your pregnancy progresses.

An HIV test may also be offered depending on which province you live in. If you are HIV positive, injections of a drug called zidovudine can greatly reduce the risk of HIV transmission to the baby.

*Urine Tests*

At most midwifery offices, the appointment begins with a urine test. You'd be amazed at the number of things you can discover by peeing on a stick! Urine is relatively simple to test using a pretreated stick or strip of paper. Pee on the stick and it will turn colour if there are elevated levels of protein, blood or sugar in your urine. You'll likely be asked to compare the colours on your stick with the sample colours that illustrate normal levels. If they differ, you'll show your stick to your midwife and she will decipher them for you and tell you if further tests are required. For example, an elevated sugar level could be a fleeting thing, or it could indicate a problem that requires attention, such as gestational diabetes. Diabetes in pregnancy can result in larger than usual babies. It can also mean there is a potential for complications such as hypoglycemia in the newborn. If your midwife suspects you have this condition, she will talk to you about the possibility of further screening.

**Testing in private**

I appreciated the fact that I was the one to check protein and sugar levels in my urine and to weigh myself. It made me feel like a competent partner in the whole business, rather than a patient.

*—Susan, mother of three*

*Blood Pressure*

The midwives will take your blood pressure at every visit. Monitoring your blood pressure during the early stages of pregnancy helps them establish a baseline for the rest of your readings. High blood pressure in pregnancy can be very serious but usually doesn't arise until the end of the second trimester. One of the complications associated with it is a condition called pre-eclampsia (also known as toxemia). Undetected, pre-eclampsia can become life-threatening for mother and baby.

## Checking On Your Baby

It's important to check on your baby as he or she grows—but how best to do that? There are several issues to consider with tests that are designed to determine the health of your baby. How invasive will the test be to you or your child? Are there potential dangers involved? What can actually be determined by the test itself: what will you know, and with what certainty, after you get the results?

Perhaps most important is this question: What will the results mean to you and the progress of your pregnancy? Your midwives will discuss with you the latest evidence-based research about certain tests and conditions. They will ask you to consider your own values, what you will do with the information, and what decisions you might be prepared to make if the results are not what you had hoped. Are there certain tests you absolutely do not want? What will you do if the preliminary tests suggest further tests may be necessary to get a more accurate diagnosis? Are there conditions under which you would choose to terminate a pregnancy?

*Listening for a Heartbeat*

The first verification that there is a separate being inside you will probably be the sound of your baby's heartbeat. First hearing it is an awesome event, one that you will have eagerly awaited. The baby's heartbeat can be detected by a pinard, a hornlike instrument often made from wood. The midwife places one end on the mother's belly, then puts her ear to the other end. The other tool midwives use is the fetoscope, which looks like a combination between a pinard and a stethoscope. Using these instruments a midwife may sometimes detect a heartbeat as early as 16 to 18 weeks. Or your midwife may have a doppler, which is a small handheld device that employs ultrasound technology. This device is more sensitive and can pick up the heart rate earlier than the other two, sometimes at around 12 weeks.

Many midwives have dopplers, but not all of them use the instruments routinely. Because the doppler relies on ultrasound technology, or sound waves, to find and amplify the baby's heartbeat, some people are cautious. There have been suggestions that not enough is known about the long-term effects of its use during pregnancy. Some midwives may therefore suggest choosing to minimize fetal exposure to ultrasound. Talk to your midwife about the use of these technologies in your care.


*Ultrasound*

Ultrasound uses sound waves that bounce around your uterus and then send back an image of your baby. An ultrasound is done at an ultrasound clinic or department in the hospital. If you have an ultrasound in early pregnancy, it may be done vaginally, but most ultrasounds involve a procedure in which the technician puts conductive jelly on the belly and then moves a smooth instrument (a transducer) over the whole belly. The ultrasound will interpret the bounces and produce a "reading," the image that appears on the screen.

An ultrasound can indicate whether the baby's organs and "structures"—the spine, palate, face, cord and so on—are developing normally. It also measures fetal size and determines the health of the placenta. In later pregnancy, the amount of fluid will also be noted. Ultrasound technology is also used to guide the needle in chorionic villi sampling and amniocentesis tests.

### Testing and personal choice

In each of my pregnancies, we chose not to do ultrasound testing. I feel that testing is an invasion of my personal space and that it is unnecessary.

We are concerned that there may be long-term health risks associated with some tests, such as ultrasound, which may not have been fully examined. Of course, the health of the baby is our primary concern. My husband and I pray about these decisions and take them very seriously. Our midwife understands our relationship with God, and her care has allowed us to make these choices in a supportive, caring environment.

—*Heather, mother of five*

### *Chorionic Villi Sampling*

Between 10 and 12 weeks of pregnancy, women are eligible for a chorionic villi sampling. In this test, some of the baby's cells developing into the placenta are extracted with a needle that is inserted through the cervix or through the stomach wall and into the uterus. The cells can then be analysed for any chromosomal abnormalities, such as Down syndrome, cystic fibrosis and muscular dystrophy. Women who have this test are at a slightly higher risk for miscarriage than those who choose amniocentesis to obtain this information.

### *Maternal Serum Screening (MSS)*

This test has become quite popular (in regions where it is available) because it is easy to do and poses no direct risks to the mother or baby. If you opt for maternal serum screening (MSS), your blood will be taken and tested sometime between weeks 15 and 17. The blood will be analysed in the lab to determine the chance of your baby having certain chromosomal abnormalities, such as Down syndrome, or open neural tube defect, which affects the spine and brain. Though this test is simple, it cannot be performed as early as chorionic villi sampling, and it is used to screen for the likelihood of abnormalities rather than to diagnose a condition in your baby. An abnormal result may lead to further testing.

### Integrated Screening and NT Screening

The detection of conditions associated with chromosomal abnormalities, such as Down syndrome and open neural tube defects, is now being improved with a two-stage test called integrated, or first trimester, screening. This test is similar to maternal serum screening in that it can be done earlier in pregnancy and poses less risk than amniocentesis. This test has a higher rate of accuracy than MSS, and results in fewer false positives.

The first stage of testing, done between 10 and 13 weeks, is a blood test and ultrasound. The ultrasound is conducted to determine gestational age, show the fetal heartbeat and measure nuchal translucency (NT), the thickness of one area at the back of the baby's neck.

The second stage of testing is another blood test, usually taken between 15 and 16 weeks, and no later than 22 weeks. The results of the two tests are then combined for a diagnosis.

Though the chance of inaccuracies is much lower with this method, there is still a possibility of false positives in the 2 percent of women who receive a positive result. In the event of a positive result, you will need to decide whether to do further testing, such as amniocentesis or high-definition ultrasound, to provide more information.

Integrated screening is a highly specialized test and is not available everywhere.

*Amniocentesis*

This procedure involves using a needle, injected through the stomach wall and into the uterus, to withdraw a small amount of amniotic fluid. The fluid contains some of the baby's cells, which can be tested in a lab for chromosomal abnormalities that point to conditions such as Down syndrome. Unlike chorionic villi sampling, amniocentesis is performed at around weeks 15 to 18 and carries a slightly higher risk of miscarriage and breathing problems at birth. Results often take two to four weeks to return from the lab.

Testing may provide you with information you feel is important for your pregnancy and your care. Still, it is wise to prepare yourself for any tests risks and results before undergoing any procedure.

**Ultrasound decisions**

My partner and I were able to choose when it was appropriate for us to do tests and have procedures done on me and the children. In both of our pregnancies, we chose not to do a routine ultrasound.

When the time came to think about the 18-week ultrasound, I decided that I didn't want to do a test just because it was routine. There hadn't been anything in my pregnancies that indicated I needed this test, so we decided to skip it. I really appreciate that my midwives respected my wishes.

*—Joy, mother of two*

*Testing for Group B Streptococcus*

In the last weeks of pregnancy, you may be offered a test for the presence of beta streptococcus, or group B streptococcus, in your vagina. Group B strep is one of the normal bacteria any woman can carry at any time, without noticeable symptoms or effects. However, if you have Group B strep while your baby makes his or her way through the birth canal, there is a risk that it can be passed to your child. Though only a small percentage of infants develop an infection, the results can be very serious and even life-threatening.

To reduce the likelihood that their babies are exposed to group B strep, many mothers opt to do a vaginal swab in late pregnancy to determine whether they are carrying the bacteria. You will probably be able to do your own swab and pass it to the midwives, who will send it to the lab.

If you test positive for the presence of group B strep, it may alter your birth plans. Though babies suspected to have come into contact with group B strep can be treated with antibiotics after birth, one recognized treatment is to give the mother antibiotics by intravenous during labour. Most midwifery clients don't intend to have an IV during the regular course of labour, and provinces have different, and changing, regulations about the use of antibiotics in a non-hospital birth place. For example, in Quebec, IVs are available at birthing centres. In Ontario, many midwives will offer IV antibiotics for a homebirth. If you test positive for group B strep, your midwives will help you determine how best to get what you and your baby need during the birth.

### Breech Babies

Throughout your pregnancy, the midwives will palpate your belly to see how your baby is growing and where he or she is lying. As you near the end of your pregnancy, the midwives will determine whether your baby is head down and secure in the birth canal, or ready to "drop" deep into the pelvis when you go into labour.

As the end of pregnancy approaches, the majority of babies will tip into a head-down position, and stay there until birth. Since head-down is the easiest way for the baby to make its way through the birth canal, the small percentage of babies that don't settle this way are often encouraged to turn.

If your baby is still facing up after 37 weeks, you may choose to have a midwife or doctor try an external version. In this procedure, your practitioner will use her hands to manipulate the baby from the outside in an attempt to get the baby head down. External versions are usually done in hospital.

Midwives' scope of practice does not generally allow them to catch breech babies, particularly without a physician in attendance. The vast majority of doctors will not consider a vaginal delivery of a breech baby, due to recent research indicating that a C-section is safer. Therefore, most parents with breech babies schedule a C-section.

## ◈ If You Want to Read More . . .

*The Complete Book of Pregnancy and Childbirth* (new ed.), by Sheila Kitzinger (London: Dorling Kindersley Limited, 1996).

*The Encyclopedia of Childbearing*, by Barbara Katz Rothman (New York: Henry Holt and Company, Inc., 1993).

*Healthy Beginnings: Your Handbook for Pregnancy and Birth* (2nd ed.), by The Society of Obstetricians and Gynecologists of Canada (Ottawa: The Society of Obstetricians and Gynecologists of Canada, 2000).

*The Mother of All Pregnancy Books: An All-Canadian Guide to Conception, Birth & Everything in Between*, by Ann Douglas (Toronto: CDG Books, 2000).

*Pregnancy and Birth: The Best Evidence*, by Joyce Barrett and Teresa Pitman (Toronto: Key Porter Books, 1999).

*What to Expect When You're Expecting*, by Arlene Eisenberg, Heidi E. Murkoff and Sandee E. Hathaway (New York: Workman Publishing, Inc., 1991).

*Your Pregnancy Week-by-Week*, by Glade B. Curtis (Tucson, Arizona: Fisher Books, 1994).

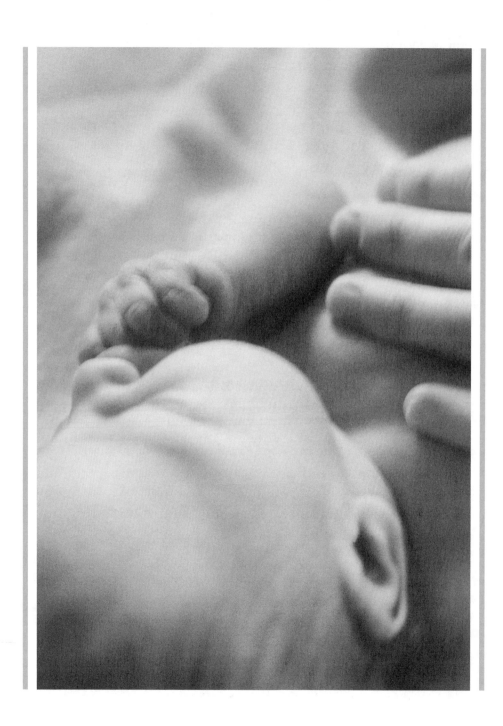

Seven

# The Birth Place

When you first contact a midwifery practice, you will probably be asked the date your baby is due and where you plan to give birth. Midwives in many parts of Canada can offer their clients a choice of giving birth at home or in hospital.

One of the many myths surrounding midwives is that they only attend homebirths. It is true that before midwifery was legislated midwives in most places were limited to aiding families who chose to have their babies at home. If circumstances required a move to the hospital, the midwife would travel with the mother, but wouldn't have any more status or influence in the delivery room than the woman's partner or mother. This continues to be the situation in many areas without midwifery legislation.

The other part of the story is that in some remote parts of Canada, midwives were actually restricted to practising only in institutions such as nursing centres. These women had dual training as midwives and nurses and were hired as nurses to practise midwifery in the hospital setting.

In the province of Quebec, the terms of legislation require midwives to attend labour in free-standing birth centres. So far, Calgary is the only place where midwives can attend women at home, in hospital or in a free-standing birth centre.

Being asked where you plan to have your baby just when you are adjusting to the concept of being pregnant, may seem a bit ridiculous. It's nine months away and you haven't yet flipped open the baby name book.

However, midwives may need this information to plan their schedules, including logistics such as how much travel time is required to get to your home for visits and possibly for the birth itself. Also, midwives in your area may be required to serve a percentage of clients at home and in hospital. In Ontario, midwives must attend at least 10 homebirths and 10 hospital births over two years to maintain their registration. As the only birth professionals who provide out-of-hospital service, midwives try to ensure that they are available for clients committed to homebirth.

So, you will be asked to tell your potential caregivers where you are thinking about having your baby. But it's important to understand that putting your hand up for a certain option does not mean that you have no flexibility. As you get to know your midwives, and they get to know you and the particular details of your pregnancy, your plans may change. For the authors' first pregnancies, both of us revised our choices as we neared our due dates. Sarah had planned a homebirth at the start, but a medical condition made it necessary for her to plan a hospital birth. Miranda had intended to have her first child in the hospital but eventually opted for a homebirth instead. So don't feel locked in. Midwives expect that your wishes may change as you begin to understand the scope of your options. If your choices are limited by complications during your pregnancy, your midwives will continue to help you find ways to plan the birth you want within the necessary parameters.

Anticipating your child's birth is a process that requires some soul-searching. Are you going to be screaming, "Give me the drugs!"? If you're at home, is your partner going to be busy washing sheets instead of snuggling with you and the baby? In the hospital, will your baby have to sleep in the nursery and be offered a bottle?

You can never know just how your birth will unfold. A certain amount of guessing and prediction are always required. Make your decisions, then allow for changes.

## Considering Hospital Birth

### The Hospital Option

Since the majority of us have not had the opportunity to witness a baby being born, most people's mental images of birth are the result of Life Network documentaries or a rerun of *Friends*. The setting for such scenes is almost always a hospital, complete with nurses yelling at the woman to "Push!"

Of course, no birth—at the hospital or at home—is just like TV. Least of all a birth with midwives.

### Labouring

Planning a hospital birth means just that: your birth will occur in the hospital. This does not mean that your entire labour, or even the majority of it, will happen there.

With first babies, labour is usually longer, and most midwives will have you divide your labour time between your home and the hospital. That way, you won't be getting there too early with nothing to do but walk the halls, and you won't be leaving home so late that your family's next generation starts life in the back seat of a car.

When you suspect you are in labour, you will call your midwife to discuss the signs. The midwives will probably not come over immediately but will stay in contact by phone. Once your labour is underway, your midwife will usually come over to assess your progress. She may advise rest or quiet activities and make plans to come back when you or your partner feel you need extra support. Of course, you and the midwives may decide that you are already at that point. Your primary midwife will help you work through the more difficult contractions, and when labour is well established and progressing, you and your midwife will make your way to the hospital. Another midwife or your midwife's second attendant will join you at the hospital in time to assist you during the pushing stage.

If you are having a very fast labour or if you need to travel a substantial distance to the hospital, you and your midwives may plan for you to leave your house quite early in labour to ensure that you get to the hospital on time. In this case, when you call, your midwife may assess your condition by phone and advise you to go straight to the hospital, where she will meet you. These plans will differ depending on whether or not it is your first baby. If you have already had children, the plans will be influenced by the length of your previous labours.

You may be labouring in three places: at home, in a vehicle on the way to the hospital, and in the hospital itself. During labour, some women enter a very internal state where the activity around them becomes insignificant or completely unnoticeable. Other mothers feel the need to concentrate and struggle to keep their focus. It is impossible to predict how busy the labour and delivery floor will be on your baby's birthday, but the midwives are very good at maintaining a sense of privacy even within the hospital.

### Preparation and Cleanup

Many of the same preparations need to be made whether you choose a home or hospital setting. You will still need to prepare your place for a new baby and for the postpartum period, and you will still have midwives coming to your home for labour and for postpartum visits. The checklist in Chapter 8 will help you get ready.

If you are having your baby in the hospital, you are saved the trouble of washing the sheets from your birth bed. Undoubtedly, this will lessen the mess factor at your home—but only by one or two loads of laundry. There is always plenty of laundry to do once the baby comes!

### Changing Your Mind

If you have planned a hospital birth, your midwives will be committed to getting you there at the appropriate time. For most people, this is very straightforward. The midwives will tell you that it will soon be time to make the trip, and they will help you get dressed or go to the bathroom and make whatever arrangements are necessary for your comfort on the way in.

Some women, however, decide during labour that they feel safer and more comfortable at home than they had expected, and start to feel that they would be happier having the baby in their own bed. At this late stage, the midwives may encourage you to go through with your pre-labour plans. You will have spent a long time considering your options, and it may be best to stick with them. If, however, you are certain about staying home, the decision—like all others—belongs to you.

### Late changes to the birth plan

When I tell people we had midwifery care and a planned hospital birth, they are very surprised to learn that we were able to do that.

Within our family, choosing to use a midwife at all was seen as something quite radical. Taking the whole step and going all the way with a midwife and a homebirth was something that my husband and I were not comfortable with and we would have had nine months of incredible pressure from our families. We also wanted to have all the medical help available should something go wrong. But philosophically, once we had taken a look at the care that we wanted and the way that we wanted to consider the pregnancy, we favoured the care and approach that comes from midwifery, where pregnancy is treated as a normal condition rather than an illness.

There was no pressure from our midwife to have a homebirth. When we first talked about our choice to have a hospital birth, it wasn't uncomfortable at all, we just continued on with the rest of the questions and the rest of the care. We didn't feel pressure at any time to consider a homebirth or to change our decision.

Much of the labour went the way we had expected. We had talked about staying home as long as possible, because at that point we were so comfortable with the midwives that we really did want to be at home for the labouring part. So we had planned to be at home until I was about seven centimetres dilated, then move to the hospital.

But when I was about three centimetres dilated, I got nervous that we wouldn't be able to get to the hospital. I don't know why, but I started worrying about the traffic, being in the car without the midwives (who had their own car), and I didn't want to be away from them for the time it would take to get to the hospital. So I asked if we could move to the hospital earlier than planned.

Once again, it was the same as any of the other decisions that we had made throughout our care. I was informed about what that change in plan would mean: how there was definitely time to move later in the labour, how being in the hospital for a longer period of time sometimes means you can't move around as much as you can at home, how I might miss the access to my own things. They made sure that I knew all of the pros and cons and that the early move was what I really wanted. As soon as I said, "This is definitely what I want to do," there were no questions asked and off we went.

I did feel better when I got to the hospital. My husband felt a lot better too. His major job was driving me to the hospital, and that job was finished. Now he could just focus on being there and helping me.

At seven centimetres, I asked for an epidural, which I got very quickly. I had about two hours of pushing, and that was it, Ethan was born!

I stayed until the next morning. I was ready to leave the hospital within three or four hours, but because my husband was so tired, we decided that he should go home and sleep. When he came back to pick me up, he had lots of energy to look after the baby and me.

—*Lisa, mother of one*

*The Hospital Environment*

You can take a tour of your local hospital to research the facilities. Keep in mind, however, that the person giving the tour may be unfamiliar with midwife-attended births. Once you have seen the space, double-check the information you received from hospital staff with your midwives and ask them about their experiences with the hospital. There may be more options available than the tour guide reveals.

Some components of the hospital environment are impossible to change: If there is only one bathroom for three birth rooms, you can't do much about it. But many elements can be modified to suit your wishes. You can dim the lights, you can play music, and you can tone down the electronic equipment—most of the time. The checklist in Chapter 8 will help you think of things to bring along to make you more comfortable.

When Sarah had her first baby at the hospital, the room was dark, quiet and relaxing. Sarah wore her own clothes but had to drape a gown over herself to go the bathroom on the other side of the hall. Before the birth she found out the beds could be lowered and shaped for her comfort. But, of course, she forgot all about that once she was in labour.

One thing the hospitals tend to be inflexible about is the burning of candles or herbs. Though this seems to be universal, if it is something you would like, ask your midwives if the hospital you are considering can accommodate your wish.

### The Stay

Even if you choose the hospital option, you will probably still spend more time at home than your friend who delivered under a doctor's supervision. If your birth is routine, your family may be ready to go home when your baby is only a few hours old.

Women under a doctor's care often have to meet specific markers before being discharged. These can be as obvious as establishing breastfeeding or as unpleasant as having a bowel movement. With midwifery care, this intensive period of observation is unnecessary. Since your midwives will visit you frequently during your first couple of days and weeks in the postpartum period and will continue to be on-call 24 hours a day, they will constantly be assessing the health of both mom and baby.

**A brief hospital stay**

We left the hospital around 6:45 A.M. The clerk couldn't believe we were in and out so quickly! It was a clear, crisp new morning and it was exciting to be out in the new day with our new son. We had seen the movie *Shakespeare in Love* a few weeks before, and there is a scene in which one character says, "It is a new day," and the heroine, who is newly in love says, "It is a new world!" That's how I felt—triumphant with the dawn. We went home, made a few phone calls, had tea and muffins and went to sleep all together in our bed.

—*Susan, mother of three*

Many families find it much easier for everyone to relax and get into a routine when they are in their own bed and surrounded by familiar people. Of course, if circumstances suggest that a longer time in hospital would be beneficial, or if you feel uncomfortable going home so soon, you can always extend your stay.

If your stay is prolonged, you will have more interactions with hospital staff than the midwifery client who goes straight home. The midwives will still make their visits and be on call for questions and reassurance of the kind you can only get from someone who knows you well.

### Safety

Many people see midwife-attended hospital births as the ultimate solution: You can have an attentive relationship with your midwife combined with access to all the modern technologies.

A hospital birth puts you closer to medical tools than does a homebirth. If you need a Caesarean, the operating room is just down the hall. Midwives don't carry Pitocin (a drug that increases the speed of labour) to homebirths nor do they perform epidurals in this setting.

But just because you're close to the tools doesn't necessarily mean you get to use them any faster. If you need a Caesarean section, staff will have to prepare the operating room and locate an obstetrician to do the procedure. An anesthesiologist is the only one who can administer an epidural, and there may be other people waiting for his or her services.

*Chances of Intervention*

One of the advantages of the Canadian system, where midwives practise in birth centres, and home and hospital settings, is that the quality of your care should not depend on the place your baby is born. Women under midwifery care should be offered the same choices regardless of chosen birth place. Many practices compare the number of interventions for their hospital and home clients. Ask your midwives about their experiences.

## Considering Birth at a Birth Centre

*The Birth Centre Option*

In Quebec and in some remote areas of Canada, choosing midwifery care automatically means one setting for your birth: the free-standing birth centre. Midwives in Quebec are legislated and funded but do not have privileges in hospitals. Provincial legislation provides for the possibility of homebirth in the future, but, as of 2002, pregnant women in Quebec were not being offered this option. In the meantime, midwives are able to offer their clients midwife-attended birth in a high-quality, home-like, institutional environment. For many women and their families, this is the perfect middle ground between home and hospital. Each of the six birth centres currently in operation is affiliated with a local community health centre.

Before parents decide whether midwifery care is for them, they take a tour of the birth centre, or *maison de naissance*, in their area. These group tours are held regularly and may be guided by a midwife or other staff member. If the woman and her support people are comfortable with what they have heard and seen, then they will book a first meeting with a midwife.

A privately owned and operated birth centre in Calgary, Alberta, is similar in look and feel to the birth centres in Quebec. The main difference is that clients who have chosen and paid for a midwife can then decide to give birth in the birth centre for an additional fee.

In some parts of Canada birth centres have been set up to support women who live in rural or remote communities and First Nations women. These centres are extremely important as they offer care to women locally and are responsive to their cultural beliefs. It is hoped and expected that additional government funding will be secured to support these important initiatives.

### Aides-natales, or Birth Attendants

Unique to the Quebec model is the *aide-natale*, or birth attendant. The role of the *aide-natale* is very similar to that of a doula: she plays a variety of roles during labour, birth and the postpartum period. The *aide-natale* may provide labour support and will be on hand to offer food and drink if needed. She also does much of the cleanup after the birth and is responsible for stocking labour rooms and sterilizing and stocking equipment. The *aide-natale* is trained to provide breastfeeding support and will also prepare and serve meals to the new mother after the birth.

### The Birth Centre Environment

If you tour your local birth centre, what you will probably see is a clean, bright environment designed to look more like a home than an institution. The clinic rooms where you have your regular visits will probably look much like clinic rooms in any midwifery practice, but the birthing rooms may be decorated with pictures and furnished with rocking chairs and a comfortable double bed. Some rooms may also have Jacuzzis for labouring in. Birthing rooms are usually set apart from the clinic space so that women can labour in privacy and families can bond in a quiet area. There is usually a larger common room or classroom for prenatal classes, yoga classes and postpartum or breastfeeding support meetings. Often there are resource libraries with books and videos in both languages. There will be a living room where support people who accompany the woman in labour can wait if the mother wants some time alone.

In addition to this space for the clients, the *maison* will have a kitchen where the *aides-natales* prepare the meals. A room with emergency supplies houses mobile incubators and medications that the midwives can administer. Administrative offices and a resting room for midwives make up the rest of the house.

*Maisons* are located in a variety of places: grand old homes attached to churches, right in the community health centre, or even in one case on the lower level of a seniors' residence. They are all similar in that they have been carefully organized and decorated to feel homelike and comfortable.

### Labouring

When you think your labour is beginning, you can call your midwife. Together you will decide when to come into the *maison*. In some cases, your midwives will arrange to meet you at home to support you in labour there. Clients are only allowed to be in labour at the *maison* for 24 hours, so take care not to arrive too early.

Your midwife will meet you at the *maison* and will stay with you through labour and into the few hours following birth. As in other places, the second midwife will be called in for the final stages of labour.

Women are encouraged to make themselves comfortable by walking, and using water or any of the other birthing aids that are available at each *maison*, such as birthing balls and birthing stools. Your midwife will help you try different techniques to move you through your labour. You are welcome to bring personal belongings, CDs and so on from home that will make you feel as comfortable as possible during labour. You may also want to bring food for your support people. (The *maison* will provide food and drinks for you during labour.)

**Having a baby at the birth centre**

I had both of my babies with midwives at a birth centre in Quebec. Initially my husband, Yves, and I considered trying to find a traditional birth attendant who would help us have our baby at home. In the end, I decided I wasn't comfortable with it because we lived at least 45 minutes away from the nearest hospital and both of our babies were born in the winter.

My first pregnancy was easy, and I developed a really great relationship with my midwife. She was very attentive, and yet if everyhting was okay she did not interfere. Late in my pregnancy I received a lot of advice from friends about things that I could do to speed things up, such as taking homeopathic remedies. I asked my midwife what she thought. She just told me, "Joy, your body is doing everything it is supposed to be doing. If you want those things, I have them and I can give them to you, but do you really need them?" That made sense to me; it calmed me down and grounded me so that I could wait for what came next.

I went into the birth centre early in my labour. My midwife had originally offered to come out to be with me at my home during my labour, but she ended up being quite busy at the birth centre that day, so we went in to meet her instead. They confirmed that I was definitely in labour, so we decided to stay.

All that night I walked and was in and out of the bath, on and off the toilet and using the bar they had to crouch. My midwife and my partner took turns sleeping and supporting me. Even in labour, I remember my midwife wouldn't really offer me advice about how to breathe or anything. She just encouraged me.

I ended up pushing for a long time. I became quite tired during this stage. When I finally pushed my baby out, they needed to work on him a bit to get him to perk up. I didn't notice any of this, but my partner was quite alarmed and couldn't even talk when our son was born. Everything was fine in the end. We got cleaned up, had a nap, and we were on our way home just three hours after our son was born.

Our midwife came to see us the next day. She spent time talking to us about our birth and our son's entry into the world. This was quite amazing. We really appreciated her insight. They helped us in "processing" the experience.

—Joy, mother of two

*Preparation and Cleanup*

At the maison, as at the hospital, all the preparations for the birthing area, and all the cleaning afterward, are handled by staff members. The systems in place to tidy up and get you settled after you have your baby are designed to minimize interruptions for the new family. You can remain in the birthing room to bond with your new baby and get some rest if you decide to stay.

### The Stay

Some women may choose to remain at the birth centre for a while after the birth. The stay can last up to 24 hours postpartum. During this period a woman may sleep, eat, shower and receive visitors. If they prefer, mothers can opt for an earlier departure. The *aide-natale* will also assist in this period to establish breastfeeding or bottle-feeding, depending on what the mother prefers.

### Midwives' Emergency Procedures and Transfers of Care

Though the birth centre is not a hospital, it will house some equipment that a midwife attending a homebirth would not have on hand, such as a mobile incubator and intravenous equipment. *Maisons* also have direct connections to ambulance services and special neonatal transport teams if the need for an emergency transport should arise.

Since midwives in Quebec are limited to practising within the *maison*, if you require transfer to hospital, the midwife will no longer be your primary caregiver. This does not mean that the midwife will leave you at the hospital door, but it does mean that your care will be taken over by a medical team. For some women, this transfer is a smooth one, and they feel reassured by their midwife's new role as a labour support person. Others, however, find the transition from the midwife approach to the medical system jarring. Like midwives in other parts of Canada, midwives in Quebec have definite standards that determine when they must transfer care to a physician. One of those instances is if labour continues beyond 24 hours.

## Considering Homebirth

*The Home Environment*

For some women, a well-appointed hospital room and the guarantee of midwifery care cannot replace the comfort of a homebirth.

A homebirth can help make having a baby feel like a truly normal occurrence. The baby emerges into the place where he or she will eat and sleep and become part of the family. In most cases, the people present are trusted and familiar individuals, and at home, distractions can be kept to a minimum.

**Jane's sense of accomplishment**

Being able to birth at home without pain relief gave me such a feeling of accomplishment and pride. I know now that I can do anything, and that power will remain with me forever.

*—Jane, mother of two*

*Company and Privacy*

If you give birth at home, the only limits on the number of people attending the birth are the ones you choose. If you want it to be just you, the baby and the midwives, that's fine. If you want your baby's birth to be witnessed by two generations of grandparents and your other kids, that's O.K. too.

But what about the neighbours? Depending on where you live, the season, and your own "volume" during labour, the neighbours may or may not be aware of the big event that's occurring at your place. Some people who live in particularly close quarters (such as apartment buildings or townhouses) prepare their neighbours during a conversation or by slipping a note under their door. We've even heard stories of neighbours who hadn't been given advance notice of a homebirth showing up a few hours later with batches of muffins.

*Homebirth Options*

At home, you don't have to worry about remembering to bring along your favourite pillow or CD because these things are all right there, at your fingertips. If you want to handle contractions in front of your fireplace or out on your balcony, go ahead. You also have the liberty of making trips to your own bathroom as undressed as you care to be.

Having your baby at home also means you can plan birthing rituals that aren't permitted at most hospitals, such as burning candles or herbs or giving birth in water. Many midwifery practices will help you make arrangements to obtain a birthing pool where you can labour and give birth.

**Cocooning at home**

When we found out we were pregnant with our first child, we lived in England but had already bought and taken ownership of our house in Toronto. It was clear we would be having the baby in Canada. I already had some experience, through my sister's births, with midwives in Ontario, so for us that was the path to take. Then came the decision of where to give birth. Without thinking about it, we had always assumed that babies should be born in hospital. Honestly, I think that at the beginning it's hard to really understand anything at all. It isn't until I was in the third trimester and really starting to understand the birth process that the decision that was right for us could be made. In the end, we decided that home was the place for us. We'd both spent time in hospitals and felt that they were places for problems and sick people, and that having a baby is normal and not necessarily problematic. I already felt that I wanted to be painkiller free, as much as possible. My theory is that my body is meant to do this and that if I can get out of my own way enough to allow that to happen, and go with it, then my body won't do anything I can't handle.

As time went on and we encountered surprised reactions from people, we began to waver a bit about our decision. So many people told us how unusual it was for a first baby to be born at home. The reality of bringing a new life into the world became daunting. Add that to the renovation we were doing on our home—dust and babies shouldn't really mix. There were a lot of considerations.

Ultimately our commitment to homebirth won out. We knew that in order to take this on we had to work together and be completely committed. We understood that there were risks associated with homebirth, but hospital birth had risks too. We chose to accept the risk associated with homebirth. We also considered other factors. We decided that we didn't like the idea of being at the mercy of hospital schedules and policies. For such an intimate experience, we wanted to be in our own home, with control over who came near us. I wanted to be completely free to do, say or scream whatever I wished. I wanted to be able to take a shower or walk around naked, all without distraction.

My husband had spent six years working as a paramedic, so I wasn't concerned about his reaction to the experience. He had also seen problems in labour and had asked the midwives a lot of questions regarding their decision-making process so that he could feel sure that if there were problems, we would be able to get to the hospital. We also pre-registered at two hospitals, just in case.

When the time came, our largest anxiety was the state of our house. We had two floors mostly renovated, with a bath and shower and some space to walk around, so it was fine in the end. Having my sister there, to take care of food and details—like phone calls and people showing up—proved essential. For the birth and for the week after, her contribution was priceless. It allowed us to be cocooned as a new family and to share our new baby with others only when we were ready.

—*Hilary, mother of two*

*Preparation and Cleanup*

Labour and birth can be a long process. Parents who plan for a hospital birth will have cafeterias and drink machines at their disposal. They will have clean sheets waiting and staff ready to mop up or cart away soiled linen.

Your home is usually a comfortable place, but keep in mind that births may take a short time or many hours. A planned homebirth requires that you have all the necessary supplies on hand, including adequate seating, food and drinks for yourself and all your attendants. The last thing you want to be doing in the early stages of labour is moving furniture or shopping.

This doesn't mean that midwives expect the Good Housekeeping Seal of Approval or that you need to create a hospital environment at home.

Some women we know have had babies in houses that are undergoing full-scale renovation. But you will need to feel confident that you have a clean place to have your baby and one in which the midwives can work well. This means preparing sheets, towels and cloths, shopping for labour aids and getting organized. Though not an awesome task (the checklist in Chapter 8 will help you), it requires a commitment.

As homebirth veterans, we will admit that the by-products of birth are messy. Amniotic fluid and baby poo make for a few dirty sheets. But it wasn't until Sarah, already a mother of two, attended the birth of her sister's child that she really noticed the mess. While the midwives don't provide a cleaning service, they will assist you by stripping the birth bed and getting you bathed and tucked in comfortably. Some midwives estimate that a homebirth amounts to one additional load of laundry and one bag of garbage. While midwives' experience has provided for lots of tips and advice that make this task much easier than you might expect, you will never love your mate, mother or friend more than when they clean up. Don't forget that they've just seen you do something difficult and amazing. Relatively speaking, their task is an easy one.

### Can You Change Your Mind?

This is a big question for many women considering homebirth. The answer is yes. If you don't feel comfortable at home, you can ask to be transferred to the hospital. You can say, "Book the epidural, I'm coming in!" Chances are, however, that your midwives will know if you're approaching this point and will offer you the option if other forms of assistance are not enough. Again, remember that midwives are about choice. They want you to feel safe and comfortable and to support you in your choices.

### Medical Assistance

Most labouring mothers who are transferred to hospital do not go there because they want pain relief, but because they know they have to in order to ensure their own safety and their baby's. Keep in mind that the vast majority of such transfers occur because labour is taking too long, not because something unforeseen occurs in a short period of time. As one of Sarah's midwives put it, "Most problems you can see coming from a long way off."

Across the country, the rates of transfer to hospital for women with planned homebirths varies. The average is about 20 percent or less, including transfers from Quebec birth centres to hospital. The majority of women are transferred because they need help to progress during a particularly long labour. In other cases a mother needs painkillers that will allow her to rest in order to avoid further interventions, such as a Caesarean.

The decision to have a homebirth can be influenced by where you live. If you are in an area with prompt emergency services and a hospital close by, it is probably going to be easier to choose a homebirth than if you are miles away from the nearest neighbour.

A smart homebirth plan makes room for the unscripted. Often your midwives will have you pre-register at your local hospital. This will minimize the paperwork if a transfer is required. If you are giving birth in an area where your midwives have no hospital privileges, you may want to consider seeing a physician occasionally during your pregnancy so that you have a name to put on the admittance form, should you need to go to the hospital. You should also know the best route to the hospital and have a phone close by, posted with emergency numbers.

In addition, you will want the midwives to check out your space. Perhaps they will suggest that one room in your home may be more conducive to the birth experience than another. Should a transfer become necessary, you need to consider whether there is enough room for a stretcher to navigate landings or elevators.

*Midwives' Emergency Procedures*

Midwives will bring standard supplies and tools to your homebirth, which will include many of the things available at the hospital. They will have oxygen for mothers and babies, tools for clearing the baby's airways, instruments for emergency episiotomies, and oxytocin injections to control excessive postpartum bleeding. In some regions, midwives can also administer antibiotics by IV.

In study after study, midwife-assisted homebirths have been shown to be a safe alternative to hospital births. Midwives can perform many emergency procedures on both mother and baby at home. However, some conditions are best treated in the hospital. If you are planning a homebirth, midwives will monitor your progress and anticipate many potential problems, allowing for time to transfer to a hospital. But in certain rare cases being in the hospital at the time the emergency arises can mean a better outcome for the mother and baby. For example, meconium staining (when baby has a bowel movement in utero) may indicate the need to transfer. Occasionally resuscitation requires drugs the midwives cannot administer at home. In some provinces, midwives' scope of practice includes intubating (inserting a breathing tube) a newborn; in others, it does not. Postpartum hemorrhage (too much bleeding after the baby is born) is serious, and is usually managed with the use of oxytocin, which the midwives carry with them. But a woman experiencing a severe hemorrhage will require hospitalization.

Choosing a homebirth means clearly considering your own ideas of risk and the birth you wish for, as well as knowing the facts about safety. Your midwife can walk you through the particulars, because she has specific knowledge of your health, history and care.


### Attitudes of Support People

How much do you care what other people think? No, really.

When awaiting the birth of their child, even the most self-reliant parents may feel vulnerable to criticism, particularly when it calls into question their concern for the newborn's safety. Just as you will find surprising allies, you will find that people from whom you expected support (or no interest at all) are all too ready to comment on the "folly" of your homebirth decision.

If the criticism comes from a colleague or a mere acquaintance, then it may be easy to ignore. If it comes from a close friend or family member, it can be hurtful and may make you question even the firmest decision to have your baby at home.

Know whose opinion you care about, then decide what to do about opposition. It is very unlikely that your birth will have an unhappy outcome. However, if your baby were to have serious complications at birth, you would probably get more support from your community if he or she were born in hospital. This would be true no matter what caused the problems and whether or not they were preventable. Can you get the unfailing support of the people you need in your corner? Can you ignore everyone else? (For more on enlisting support, see Chapter 3.)

## Making Your Decision

Some people find that choosing their child's birth place takes a lot of time and consideration. One morning you may be certain that your baby should be born at home, but by evening you may feel committed to giving birth in hospital. Changing your mind like this is quite normal and means you are considering your options fully. Even if you are very clear about where you want to have your baby, or if circumstances dictate where you must give birth, it takes time to visualize your baby's birth in a prescribed setting.

### Making decisions as partners

Choosing where to have our baby was something my husband Ihor and I did together, which was great. After the prenatal classes, I wanted to have the baby at home. We were excited because no one else we knew had decided this. Then I got scared, and started to change my mind. But Ihor said, "I still think a homebirth would be fine, but you have to feel good about it."

We worked out this decision in a way that we don't usually work things out together. I wouldn't have gone through that whole process with Ihor if I had just gone to an obstetrician. With midwifery care we had to choose and we had to talk about our choices. The talking about it, the feeling like it was a decision we could make together, that was good for us. I felt so good about him when he supported me in what felt comfortable to me.

—*Jessica, mother of two*

The best reasons to plan a home or hospital birth are your particular circumstances and your comfort level. Your assessment should be based on where you really feel safe and comfortable—not where you believe you *should* feel safe and comfortable. Having an environment that feels secure to you will aid your labour immeasurably. One midwife told us that there can be a big difference between what people *think* about birthing at home or in hospital and what they *feel*. Try to get to the heart of your feelings, and be honest with yourself.

Don't worry about what your midwives will think about your choice or assume that they are biased toward one location or another. The midwives' role is to help ensure that parents are well informed about their choices and make decisions that suit them. With this big choice, as with all the others you'll encounter, you can consider the options available to you and the advice and recommendations of your midwife about your specific care. Once you make your choice, you can, and should, expect full support.

## ◎ *If You Want to Read More . . .*

*Birth Your Way: Choosing Birth at Home or in a Birth Centre*, by Sheila Kitzinger (London: Dorling Kindersley Limited, 2001).

*The Complete Book of Pregnancy and Childbirth* (new ed.), by Sheila Kitzinger (London: Dorling Kindersley Limited, 1996).

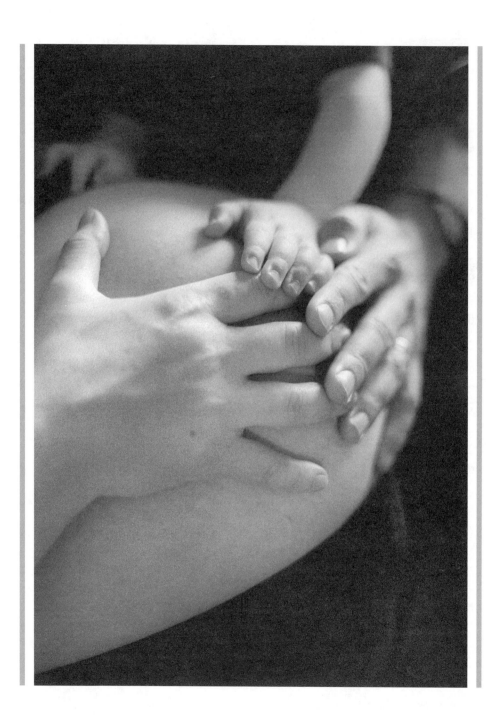

Eight

# Choosing Your
# Labour Support People

In the birth rituals of most societies, a formal social convention dictates who attends a child's birth. In some cultures, birth is viewed as a private event between a woman and her baby; in others, a labouring mother will be attended by a variety of women from her community and perhaps also her father and grandfathers.

In some rural and remote parts of Botswana, for example, it is considered ideal for a woman to go into the bush beyond her village to labour and give birth to her baby alone and in silence. First-time mothers who are unable to meet their goal of a solitary experience are attended by mothers, sisters or aunts. In Hawaii, labouring in the presence of close friends and family is so important that a woman may place a rock outside the doorway to symbolize those who are missing. In many Tibetan villages the whole community assists in the birth. This is an extremely important rite of passage not only for the mother and the baby but also for young girls, who will someday go through the same ritual. Tibetan men and boys are part of the birth as well, helping out or performing ritualized activities around the birth. The event of a birth is seen as a training ground for everyone.

In Canada, by the middle of the twentieth century, those who attended women at births were almost exclusively medical professionals, and often strangers to the mother and her family. Family members and friends were usually kept away from the labour and delivery room, and left to pace the hospital halls or sent home to await a phone call. Today, all mothers assume they will be allowed the company of at least one family member or friend.

In Canada, the range of what women want for their birth experience is almost endless, and many can be accommodated with midwifery care. Most women choose to be supported by a partner or a close friend or family member; some choose to include several generations of their family in the moment when the new child arrives. Other women labour with just the midwives present or choose to labour in solitude, with midwives and family close by. Yet we also know of people who have staged entire party-like events for their labour and their baby's arrival.

So who should be at *your* birth? Whoever *you* want or need to be there. And that could be the end of the chapter, except that the decision is not always so easy. Decisions about who should be the family birth attendants can be loaded with significance. There are many stories of grandmothers arriving at the labour room uninvited, knitting in hand, ready to survey and comment on the event.

The ability to control your birth environment is one of the reasons many women embrace midwifery care. The people around you form a significant part of that environment. You may want the birth to be completely private and have only your partner and midwives to help you through it. You may believe that involving your larger circle will enrich the experience for you, your baby and your support people too. If you plan carefully, considering your personality and your relationships, either scenario or something in between can be arranged.

## Qualities in a Labour Support Person

Here are questions to think about when considering who might be at your birth:

### Can You Count On Them to Come?

You can book an appointment for a C-section, you can book an appointment for an induction of labour, but you cannot book a time for a birth. A support person has to be available when the baby is ready, and that could be at 2:00 A.M. during a snowstorm, or in the midst of a birthday party or a big meeting. If you are counting on someone to be present for your labour and the baby's birth, determine their flexibility and commitment.

### Do They Want to Be There?

Even the most loving grandmother or trusted friend may not be prepared to witness the birth process. Some grandmothers feel that being present while their granddaughter deals with the pain of labour may be too overwhelming. If someone you would like to be present feels that he or she is not a good candidate, learning more about birth and your expectations of labour may help him or her adjust to the idea. Sometimes a solution is to have these reluctant witnesses nearby while you are labouring so that they can choose to come in if they feel comfortable at the time. If, however, their fear or discomfort is too great, it is best to respect that feeling. The centre of attention at your labour should be you and the work you are doing, not a frightened or unwilling observer.

### Are You Totally Comfortable with this Person?

Birth is a naked moment. This can be true in a literal sense as hot flashes often make wearing clothing uncomfortable. But it's also true in a figurative sense, even if you remain robed from head to toe. For during birth you use your strength and reveal your fears and other emotions. It is not a time to feel self-conscious.

Some of us feel quite comfortable revealing ourselves to those around us, while others reserve that for only a few people. If you are not willing, or able, to "let go" in front of someone, then he or she will probably not be a help in labour and may actually hinder your confidence and ability to birth your baby.

### Will They Give You Appropriate Support?

Your support people are there to help you do your best, which you are quite capable of doing. Like your midwives, they need to see you as strong and up to this task.

> **Supporting a friend in labour**
>
> When Petra was born, I was looking after her two brothers in the room next door. I talked to them and reassured them that Mommy was fine and kept them posted on what was going on. I really loved how the midwives just came into the house and facilitated things without taking over. It seemed to me a mundane miracle that all of a sudden there was a baby in the room, but it was the most normal, "doable" thing—because Caroline did it.
>
> —*Tracy, mother of one*

This includes recognizing your choices. You have chosen your midwives for their approach, skills and support, and the people who attend your birth need to respect your choice and understand the midwives' role and abilities. They need to recognize your relationship to the baby's other parent and realize that this is primarily an experience for the two of you. If you are having your baby at home, the people at your home need to approve of that choice.

People who give support during labour need to be skilled at taking direction or anticipating your needs. Many times, a labouring mother will want the physical presence of another person as she experiences contractions—perhaps to rub her back, to breathe with her, or just to be nearby. If there are a number of people at the birth, however, she probably won't want to be stared at by a panel of observers while she works through every contraction. If your partner is holding you up and walking with you, other support people can take cues from both of you about what might be needed next. Are you thinking about heading for the tub? They can make sure it is hot when you get there. Is the phone constantly ringing? They can turn off the ringer so you can concentrate (ask them to remember to turn it back on later!). Are mealtimes passing by unnoticed? They can lay out food so that everyone can keep up their strength. The key is for them to provide this support without a lot of commotion so that you are unaware of the effort involved. You will have enough to think about.

### Private labour, public birth

When I was about five months pregnant, we decided to have a homebirth. Almost as soon as we made the decision to do this, we thought that it would be great to give other friends and family members the opportunity to be there too. A birth is not something they'd get to see every day.

So when we told people we would be having a homebirth, we invited them to attend at the same time. They all thought we were nuts. Both sets of parents said, "No way! You can tell us about it when it's over and that will be just fine." I think they were really terrified that something might go wrong. But some people said yes, right away. My husband Ian's two brothers and my sister-in-law Jen said they'd like to be part of it. One friend of ours took a little bit longer to decide. Then he phoned us and said he'd like to be there. He happens to be a photographer, and he offered to take pictures.

My water broke somewhere around midnight on a Sunday night two and a half weeks before my due date. It wasn't a gushing break. It was a little leak, so I went back to bed, with no contractions, and didn't say anything to anybody. I got up the next morning and went to work. At around 8:00 A.M., I had my first contractions, but they were very light.

I called the midwives at noon. They suggested that I come over so that they could check me. They assessed the situation and suggested that I go home to rest. I made my way home, with a few stops along the way to pick up the rest of my homebirthing supplies, and called my husband to tell him what was up. He came home at about 7:00 P.M., and I called my sister-in-law and brother-in-law, who came over at 8:30 P.M., prepared to stay over.

I went into a separate room as I felt I needed my quiet space. I sort of told everyone to stop talking to me. I said I was fine and that when I needed them I would tell them, but for now I just wanted them to go away. We've known each other for a long time and I'm a straightforward person, so they understood. They would come in and check, but they basically left me alone. My sister-in-law stayed up with me all night while my husband and her husband went to bed. It's not like we sat and talked, because by the time she arrived the contractions were pretty strong and I really couldn't talk during them. She was just kind of quiet.

The midwives came to check me during the night, but I had only dilated about three centimetres. We all knew it was going to be a long haul, so they left to get a few hours of sleep, planning to return at around 9:00 A.M.

As I laboured all the next day, I kept myself in a very dark room. The midwives checked on me once in a while and my husband and Jen would come up to see if I needed anything. I felt more comfortable sitting and relaxing and going with the flow than talking. I was tired and I wanted to be alone in order to concentrate on my breathing.

My husband's brothers and our friend were sitting downstairs and were getting a little nervous because it was taking so long. Although the midwives were telling them what was happening, they really didn't have a clue.

Finally, in the late afternoon, I was ready to push the baby out. We had set up the downstairs living room as the birthing room. We had a blow-up air mattress on the floor and garbage bags over the carpeting, and we had a couch at the far end of the room for the three guys when the time came. When the baby was starting to crown, we called everyone in. They crept around the corner, quiet as mice. I was joking around at this point and just said, "Come on in! You can sit over there!" They looked nervous, as if they wondered what they were getting themselves into.

I was in a squat facing them. My husband was sitting on a chair behind me and holding me between his legs. About 15 minutes later, our son was born. Everyone got to watch, and we took pictures while it was all happening.

As you can imagine, we've talked about it since on a number of occasions. What

I remember was everyone's sense of awe. They were talking more among themselves than to me. They said things like, "Wow! That was really cool!" and "I didn't really know what to expect." My sister-in-law was quiet and bawling her eyes out. My husband had tears in his eyes, and I was thinking, Wow. Cool. There's my baby. They all stayed in the room while the midwives checked the placenta, and I heard all the people we'd invited saying, "That's so cool!"

We phoned everybody when the baby was born and both sets of parents came over. They made dinner for us because everybody was starving by then. I went to bed with the baby at 10:30 P.M., and they stayed up till about 1:00 A.M. I think they all had their own things to say about how they felt while they were waiting for the baby to be born.

I can't think of anything better than sharing a birth with family members. They will remember this for the rest of their lives. Later, everybody who had been to the first birth, plus everyone who had turned down our invitation to attend, decided to be there when we had our next baby—even our parents. When the baby ended up coming too fast for even the midwives to get there, they were really disappointed they had missed it.

*—Janine, mother of two*

### Can You Count On Them to Leave?

When they have their babies, animal mothers go alone to a quiet place away from all distraction. However, humans usually feel safer in the company of others. Many studies show that women who are accompanied by a supportive person during labour and birth have fewer interventions, require less pain relief and feel more satisfied with the outcome of their labour and delivery. Most labours are not wall-to-wall cheering but rather involve a combination of quiet time alone or with your closest support person, and time with your midwives and possibly a larger group of supporters. If you need more quiet during labour, for a short time or a long time, your support people need to be ready to make a quick exit, without a lot of prompting or commotion and without taking offence.

### How Might They Deal with the Unexpected?

Though labour is a process with specific stages, all women labour differently. You may be a very quiet person, but you may find that you need to vocalize a lot during your labour. Your personal support people need to be able to deal with who you are during labour, even if that is different from what they, or you, expected.

Births rarely go exactly as planned, and often minor alterations go unnoticed. Sometimes, however, bigger changes in thinking or action are required. If your planned homebirth unexpectedly involves transfer to hospital, how will your potential support people handle the change? In the rare case that emergency action is required, will they be able to help you stay calm and strong?

### Will They Be Willing to Educate Themselves?

Anyone you ask to be present at your birth should be prepared for the sights and sounds of the experience. An uneducated support person may be frightened by the intensity and length of labour, even when it is going well. He or she may transfer that fear to you or other support people in the room. Make sure anyone who plans to be there is well-informed and understands that the birth process takes a great deal of effort and time. They should also know about your particular preferences, concerns and hopes.

When Sarah asked her sister Hilary to attend the birth of her second child, they were living on different continents. Taking her sister to prenatal classes or midwife appointments was out of the question. Still, Hilary was able to read about the birth process and discuss Sarah's hopes and fears by phone and e-mail, which made her a confident helper when the time came.

### Will This Person Add to Your Birth Experience?

Keep in mind that most of the baby's and the mother's work occurs when the baby is still inside. You will probably be impatient for labour to end, but it's important that the other people in the room do not feel this way. Birth is usually a long process, and trying to speed it up without good reason is a dangerous thing to do. The midwives will help you labour as your body needs to. Adding someone who wants to "get to the good part" and isn't interested in the work you're doing could make you feel rushed and incompetent.

If the witness will not likely understand this, but you feel that it is important for him or her to see the baby when it arrives, you may want to consider having that person close enough to be summoned when the baby is crowning or when the baby is just a few minutes old. This is often a good plan for younger children, as well as for goal-oriented adults. Or you may choose to remind this person that the baby's life should be a long and full one, and that there will be plenty of time to bond with the newborn when things have settled down a few days after the birth.

The type of person most likely to support you during labour is:

- Someone who respects your choices
- Someone who can support you and your partner
- Someone who can take care of himself or herself
- Someone who can handle seeing you in pain.

The type of person most unlikely to support you is:

- Someone who needs directions and attention
- Someone who reacts badly under pressure
- Someone who does not acknowledge the midwives' role
- Someone who is not confident that you can have a "natural" birth.

## Partners at the Birth

Not every woman has a partner and not every woman's partner is able to be or interested in being part of her labour and the baby's birth. This can be hard to accept in a society where every TV sitcom has a father rushing to his wife's side, just as 30 years ago they paced halls and handed out cigars. If you will not have a partner with you as you labour and give birth, make sure that another friend or family member is available to support you if you wish it.

One of the fears that male partners, and female partners too, sometimes express about midwifery care is that they will be left without a role during the pregnancy and the birth. Midwifery care is woman-centred care, but it is also family-centred care. Midwives respect the relationship between you and your partner, and know that the birth of your child is a significant event in your lives together. Midwives realize that they have a limited role in helping to build your new family and that at some point you will be "on your own." Far from obstructing or ignoring the partner's place in pregnancy and birth, midwives support the family as a whole, and that means they listen to and look after both both parents.

### A dad's support

One of Lorraine's biggest fears was the labour itself. She woke at midnight with her water breaking, and the beginning of her labour seemed manageable. However, in the morning her progress seemed to stall, but she was still in a lot of pain. She was tired and discouraged. Our midwife told me we would need to go to the hospital soon for additional help. She suggested we go into the shower and not get out until the hot water ran out. It was there that I probably made my most significant contribution to my wife's labour.

Lorraine told me that she couldn't take it anymore and felt ready to give up. I asked her if she trusted our midwife and she said yes. I told her our midwife had said things were not progressing as well as they should, but that both she and the baby were still in good shape. I was honest with her. I told her that if things did not progress in the shower, then we would need to go to the hospital, but there was no shame in that. I told her I had absolute faith in her and believed in her strength.

In the shower, the contractions began to come fast and furious. I was absolutely amazed that Lorraine could stand the pressure and obvious discomfort she was in. We got out of the shower and the midwife and midwifery student checked Lorraine. She was at nine centimetres and we were back in business. Our midwife told me the "rah rah" speech I had given Lorraine was the perfect mix of compassion, caring and strength.

An hour or so later, Lorraine felt ready to begin pushing. She tried pushing in every position possible. She pushed lying on her side. She pushed lying on her back. She pushed standing up. She pushed squatting on something that looked like a milking stool. She pushed on all fours. Lorraine was becoming exhausted. We all knew that if we waited any longer, she might not be able to push the baby out. We went to the hospital.

After an 18-hour labour, Lorraine gave birth to a beautiful and healthy baby girl named Jocelyn, with a little help from a vacuum extraction. I was thrilled to have the privilege of cutting the cord and being the first to hold her. For the first time since Lorraine became pregnant, I was more than support for my wife: I had become an integral part of this new unit called a family.

*—Russ, father of two*

Partners who have been present at prenatal classes or midwifery appointments are more likely to understand their role in the labour and birth, even if they feel somewhat frightened by the prospect. Talking to you and the midwives will clarify for your partner what to expect in labour and birth and ways he or she can help during labour. Many women say that it was nothing specific that their partners did during labour that made their contributions significant. The important thing was their presence and the way they expressed confidence in the work the mothers were doing.

Some partners feel intimidated by the prospect of seeing blood or by the idea of seeing their loved one in pain. And some women express concern that their partner will not be able to see them as a sexual being after watching them give birth. In Brazil, which has one of the highest Caesarean section rates in the world, this is a commonly held belief and women often choose to forgo the support of their partners or opt for a C-section rather than have their partners witness a vaginal birth. In our experience and in the stories we have heard from women around the country, this concern vanishes during the actual labour and birth. The intensity of the birth experience and the opportunity to be together to watch your child being born become all-encompassing. In our experience, even partners who were initially reluctant observers came out of the experience saying they wouldn't have missed it for the world and felt awe-inspired by the work women do in labour. We have heard many people say they gained a new respect for their partners when they saw the enormous amount of strength required to birth a baby, whether that birth was straightforward and short or whether it involved 30 hours of labour followed by a C-section. Feeling supported, feeling confident in your partner's abilities is a great way to dive into your role as new parents or as parents of an expanded family.

## Grandparents at the Birth

Your mother or your partner's mother may be a natural choice for your personal support person, and many grandmothers today witness their grandchildren's births. If your mother (or father or parent-in-law) is your confidante and your biggest fan, and if she respects your choices as well as your relationship with your partner, this could be a wonderful experience for you all.

Keep in mind that many women who are now becoming grandmothers had a very different experience of birth than the one you are planning with your midwives. For many mothers, particularly in North America, birth was a highly medicalized event. In some cases women were even put to sleep for vaginal births and thus have no recollection of their children coming into the world. Women usually gave birth on their backs and in stirrups, or, sometimes, strapped to the delivery table. Women often laboured alone for hours and were shaved in the name of sterility.

If this was your mother's experience, she may well applaud your choice to do things differently. But she may also have lingering fear over the experience and be less likely to trust your body's abilities and your midwives' skills. Your mother may benefit a great deal from visiting the midwives with you and from talking to them and to you about her experiences. This will allow her to address in advance any fears or assumptions she has about the birth before your labour starts.

Some new mothers report a wonderful transformation in their parents' beliefs about birth, which stems from the experience of witnessing their daughter's labour and their grandchild's birth in a calm and supportive environment. Miranda's father didn't witness his grandchild's homebirth, but he was in the house and came into the room as soon as he heard the baby cry. Later he was overheard saying, "This is the way it should be done."

When you are in the process of choosing support people, it is a good idea to consider why you want them at the birth. This is especially true for parents. Even when we are adults our parents exert a huge influence on us and our behaviour, and you don't want to be worried about seeking approval during labour. Choose each person you invite for what you feel he or she can add to the experience, not because it is the conventional thing to do. Your sister may have asked your mother to her birth, your friends may have asked theirs, but if your mother is unlikely to be an appropriate support person *for you* in labour, if there are issues between your mother and your partner, if she is concerned about the choices you have made about your birth, then her presence is likely to influence the experience in a negative way. In this case it would be better to give her other responsibilities to keep her feeling involved.

### A grandmother's story

When I was invited to participate as a support person in the birth of the child expected by my son Mike and his wife, Myriam, I felt it was a great privilege. Having delighted in the three previous birth experiences I had had with two stepdaughters, both of whom had chosen midwives and homebirths, I felt sure I knew what to expect. For weeks, I had been packed and ready to bolt from work. I had comfortable clothes and a list of food to bring for all involved. I had stocked the freezer with soups and had bags of ice chips on hand. The camera was charged, and I had even taken out some long-forgotten knitting for those less calm moments.

How convenient it turned out to be: A call came only two days after the due date, and on a Friday, when leaving the office would not pose problems for me. The whole weekend lay ahead, and I could spend time doing whatever was needed. This was to be a very thoughtful baby.

In Quebec, midwives work out of birth centres, so the rendez-vous was with the Centre de Naissance in Gatineau. A fine old house. In an earlier life, it had been a priest's house. It had front and back staircases and lots of high ceilings and appropriate space for labouring and for waiting. It helped me that Mike and Myriam had been very clear beforehand about my role and what they needed by way of support. Myriam knew she would prefer to labour privately with her partner. She thought her mom could spell Mike off at times. My role was to support Mike throughout, be there for them both, and to supply food. This meant I must be patient, and that I would be part of the birth when that time arrived. I was glad to be part of it and pleased that Mike and Mimi knew what they wanted.

It was hard, however, not to feel more useful as the hours stretched on. I bolted up every time the wonderful midwife wafted by, to see if any reports could be shared. Fortunately, the birthing centre had a guest room with two sofas, where the two expectant grandmothers and Julie, Myriam's sister, could spread out. We got some sleep on Friday night. We were the lucky ones. Mike and Myriam laboured on. By Saturday morning, we were beginning to feel quite anxious. But we still felt optimistic as the midwives assured us all that it was progressing and that Myriam was doing very well. Mike appeared periodically, looking exhausted. He ate a little, then went back in quickly to offer support. He was feeling that he could not do enough, although he knew that Mimi felt comforted by his presence.

Over the course of Saturday, we listened to another mother giving birth, with lots of noise and clatter. I kept offering food to whoever came by in a futile attempt to keep busy. Even the knitting I had brought came in handy, despite the fact that I had not knitted for three years, as I had already read through my reading material. Eventually, the knitting was shared by Mary, Myriam's mom, in an effort to do something productive. As before, we both jumped up at the first hint of some new information. We were hungry as could be for news of the impending birth, but worried that things were not going easily for Mimi.

By early evening, it was clear that transfer to the hospital was a real possibility. A call to my stepdaughter, who is close to the birthing scene, proved comforting, as she reminded me of other "long labours" and reassured me that nature would take its course.

When news came that it was necessary for Myriam to go to the hospital, there was a moment of deep discouragement and concern. As support people, we had not been feeling very useful, and it was hard to really understand why things were moving this way. The midwives took time to explain the reasons to us, and that was very helpful. As we packed up, our thoughts were only with Myriam and how she would manage a car trip after all that incredible effort over 24 hours. Manage she did—she even cracked a joke here and there. We were so impressed. Once we arrived at the hospital, the atmosphere seemed impersonal. However, as the staff attended to Myriam, it was clear that the nurses were going to be terrifically supportive; the midwife who had travelled with us was also a great comfort.

The best part of the support role is getting to the birth. For me, watching and being part of the final moments is a thrill, although it is also very difficult to watch the effort needed. Holding Myriam's leg, as a contraction led to a push and deep breaths to move the baby forward, was like giving her some of my strength and feeling some of her courage.

And there, at last, was Liam, a long and healthy baby. He looked peaceful and ready to gaze out at this wondrous person who had toiled so hard to bring him into the world. There was a radiant look of wonder, satisfaction and love from Myriam and Mike that wiped away the past 30 hours of labour. I cried. I felt so connected to this child, his parents and to the world of women who bring life forward with so much love.

—*Martha, mother of two, stepmother of five, grandmother of seven*

## Friends and Family

If you called either of us in the middle of the night to say you were in labour, we'd both be in the car half dressed a minute or two later and ready to drive across town. Maybe we're a little weird that way. But many other people are not so keen on witnessing the experience. When Miranda considered whether she would have anyone aside from the midwives and her husband present at the birth of her first child, she realized her closest friends probably would not want to be there. They'd supported her through everything, but they would draw the line at birth. One of them didn't even want to go out with Miranda as her due date neared, fearing Miranda would go into labour and that she would be a surprise witness to the event!

But you may have sisters, brothers, cousins or friends whom you would like to invite to the birth and who are up for the event. Anyone who has never attended a birth will need a good introduction to the experience, which they can get from books, videos, your prenatal classes, or by going with you to an appointment with your midwives.

Women who are mothers need to understand your choices too, and respect them. Whether or not they are familiar with the midwifery model of care, they need to understand that your birth will not be the same as their experiences. If they laboured for 40 hours and then had a C-section, they need to know that this is not the way birth always happens. If they are attending your birth, they must respect your decisions to try for a birth without interventions, even if they experienced almost no pain by opting for an early epidural. No one should come to a birth with an "I told you so" attitude—unless it is "I told you you could do it!"

### Support in changing circumstances

When I became pregnant I didn't have many friends with children, and knew only one other couple that had used a midwife. While my partner MaryLou and I quite liked the idea of having midwives deliver our baby, we were still undecided until we had our first visit. At that visit, all of our questions were answered and the myths we held about midwifery were dispelled. In retrospect, I can't imagine not having chosen midwives. Throughout both my pregnancies and after our babies were born the care they provided was so personal and attentive. While the primary reasons we chose midwifery had to do with the physical and emotional care I would receive throughout the pregnancies, it was also important to us that my partner was seen and dealt with completely as my partner and co-parent of these babies. I knew what it was like to have to conceal the nature of my relationship in some of the work I did, as at times it most certainly threatened my job security. I did not want to face the possibility that either our relationship or MaryLou's role as a parent would be seen as less legitimate than a heterosexual union. With our midwives, we were fully respected as a couple.

At the outset of my pregnancy we had planned a hospital birth, but that isn't how it turned out. I went into labour ten days early and had only finished working the day before. I had a cold, a broken toe, and was feeling rather unprepared for childbirth. We had missed the prenatal class on "Labour" and hadn't quite managed to read that chapter in the book yet. However, it didn't seem that our little one cared much about any of that. He was ready to come out and it was clear that, for the first of a million times, he would have the final say.

My contractions began well before dawn on a Friday morning. I waited until the sun was fully up to call my sister Debbie, who was planning to fly in from the States for the birth. We told her that we weren't sure if this was a "false alarm", but she said she would come anyway and would arrive late that night. Mild contractions continued all day and I maintained phone contact with my midwife throughout. Late Friday evening it became clear that this was really 'it' and everyone began arriving around midnight. I remember the serenity of my bedroom where I laboured all night—one small dim lamp in the corner and quiet throughout the house—an atmosphere created by my midwife. MaryLou, Debbie and I were in the bedroom most of the night, and in the wee morning hours I even managed to doze a bit between contractions. My midwife slept in a room nearby and came in frequently to check on me and the progress of my labour. She blended in seamlessly with the calm and I hardly noticed her presence, although I felt immediately comforted and reassured every time I saw her gentle, smiling face.

When the sun began to pour through our bedroom window on Saturday morning my midwife suggested that we could speed up the process if my waters were broken. She also said that it would be a good idea to move to the hospital as planned before we did this. It struck me in that moment that I hadn't thought about that transfer even once throughout the night. The very idea of getting dressed, making my way downstairs and into a car on this cold wintery day, in the midst of contractions, was almost enough to make me want to forget about having the baby altogether. I couldn't believe that this was the time that most women transferred to the hospital! I asked if it was too late to change my mind and have the baby at home. My midwife laughed, saying this wasn't really the preferred time to be making this decision. Nevertheless, she felt that she knew us well enough to trust our decision. My labour was going smoothly and we had discussed the possibility of a home birth in the preceding months, so she sent the student midwife off to get the additional items needed for a home birth.

As we carried on at home, my mother called in for an update. I remember hearing my sister engage in a long conversation with her about why I was all of a sudden having a home birth. When Debbie told her I was too tired to go, my mother insisted that we call an ambulance to take me to the hospital. I remember thinking then that it was a good decision not to have my mother at the birth.

At 11:30 A.M. David was born into our lives. After the midwives left, MaryLou, Debbie and I spent the next few hours totally enraptured with our new little miracle.

David's birth had gone so well that we planned a home birth when I got pregnant again. Our daughter, Liora, was born three years later—same scene, nearly the same cast, (we had additional support—two friends spent the night when I went into labour to be there and help care for David.) After a labour lasting nearly as long as his own, David witnessed the birth of his sister and touched her toes just moments later.

*Paula, Mother of two*

## Doulas at the Birth

In some parts of Canada, doulas, or professional labour support people, are becoming a popular inclusion in the birth process. Doulas can be highly skilled at educating women about birth and providing emotional support during labour. They are a huge blessing for many women who are having a physician-assisted birth and want to avoid interventions. They are also enormously helpful to women who feel they need additional personal support. Doulas will often spend a great deal of time with the family before and after birth.

Doulas are not mini-midwives and do not provide the kind of clinical care that midwives do. They are professionals in their own right and offer a different kind of supportive care. Some women choose to add them to their circle of birth support people, even if they have chosen midwifery care. One woman told Sarah that her husband wanted her to hire a doula to provide the kind of support to her that he felt he couldn't.

Doulas are contacted, hired and paid for by you and may provide a range of supports, such as prenatal classes, labour support and postpartum care, including breastfeeding support and light housekeeping. Some may provide only one of these services or a combination. Asking other mothers and consulting listings online or in the Yellow Pages may help you find a doula that offers the types of services you want.

### A quiet observer

When his sister was born, my son came to the birth centre along with a friend of the family to keep him company. In the end, he sat on his daddy's lap and watched the whole thing. He was so still and quiet while he watched the baby crown. He was completely fascinated by it all! After the baby and I got cleaned up, my son and his dad went for a "swim" in the tub and all four of us curled up for a nap. We had planned to stay the whole 24 hours, but a big snowstorm was brewing, so we packed and headed for home. It ended up being just perfect.

*—Joy, mother of two*

## Children at the Birth

Miranda thought that having children at a birth was an insane idea, until a quick first labour and an extremely late call to the midwives meant that one of the midwives who could arrive most quickly had her five-year-old in tow. The little girl's mother had been a midwife since before she was born, but the girl had never witnessed a birth herself. She was safely stowed downstairs watching a video until Miranda and her husband invited her to come up to watch. She was a quiet and calm observer, and her presence seemed to give the whole event an extra significance.

Having children at the birth is not for every mother or for every child, but when everyone is comfortable with the idea it can be an amazing way to involve the whole family. The key is to find a way for everyone to feel good about the experience.

### A child's perspective

I remember when Linda [my stepmother] was first having her baby. It was early in the morning. I don't know what time, I just know it was early. I woke up and saw the midwives coming to the house. When I woke up, I saw Uncle David. Then I noticed that my brother Josh was already awake. Then I heard noises coming from the other room. Not loud noises, just sounds. I went over and saw Linda having her baby. Midwives were helping Linda. One was telling her to breathe and the other to push. Dad was beside her talking to her. Then he went and helped the midwives and talked with them about something. I went back into the other room and waited a couple of minutes. Dad called me in when the baby was pushed out. Linda was holding the baby, then I got to hold him. Then Josh came in and it was his turn. The baby's cord was still attached to his belly button. I had never seen that before. I remember the baby crying after he came out. He cried a long time. I was glad that I got to be there for all this.

—*Jeremy, age six, brother of two*

First of all, you need to acknowledge that a child is really strictly an observer, not a support person in the same way as an adult. Even older children can be overwhelmed by the intensity of birth, and children should not be asked to put aside their needs to meet the greater needs of the labouring mother. A snack *right now* is a very important thing to a three-year-old, and a child has no way to compare it with the intensity of your contractions and your need to concentrate on those.

So that you can focus on labour, so that your partner can focus on you, and so that your child can still feel safe and cared for, a trusted friend or family member should be devoted solely to the child during labour. This person needs to understand and accept his or her role; the child, in turn, needs to enjoy this person's company enough that their spending an extended amount of time together is something to look forward to. That person can care for your child while you labour, and then be responsible for bringing in your child when you are ready. For many families, this means right as the baby is crowning.

As we've mentioned, anyone who has never seen a birth before needs some education, particularly children. Grown-ups often think that blood or noise may disturb children, but often kids are fine with the things we think will faze them, and scared by things we never anticipated. If you plan to have your children at the birth, make sure you and your partner talk to them about what to expect. Give them some examples of the sounds you might make and the way you might look during labour. Show them films and books about what a baby looks like as it grows and how it comes out, and talk to them about the hard work involved. You will also want to make room for the unscripted. If you require an unexpected intervention, your child will probably not be allowed to stay with you. If you have a fast birth at 3:00 A.M., you may opt to let your child sleep through it. If you give birth suddenly during the day, there may be no time to get him home from school. It's a good idea to talk about what you would like to happen but not to make any promises.

### Sisters

Right after the baby was born, we woke up the girls and I took a shower. When I came out, I asked Richard and the midwives, "Umm, where's the baby?" I looked and there were Claire and Mali sitting in a big chair with Liz right in their lap. Liz was looking up at them and they were looking down at her. They were in this love-in for 20 minutes, at 3:00 A.M. after we had had this beautiful baby.

—*Janet, mother of three*

Make sure that in planning whether to have your children at the birth, you also ask them whether they want to be there. If they don't, then it is best to respect their wishes. Even kids who seem very keen on being part of their sibling's birth may not want to be in the room when the time comes. If there is a neutral zone within your house or the birthing centre or hospital, then kids can keep their options open and perhaps change their minds.

### A family birth day

The day of my second child's birth was scorching hot, and there was very little air moving through our bedroom in the attic of our apartment. I woke up and realized that I felt quite unwell. I woke my husband to tell him. He immediately suggested he call work to tell them the baby was coming and that he wouldn't be in that day. This pattern—the hot, hot day, and feeling bad the moment I woke up—echoed the circumstances on the day my first child was born. But I didn't feel quite as bad as I had when I had Evie. Even though I had started losing my mucous plug the day before, I didn't want Jordan to miss a day of work. He was allowed exactly two weeks' holiday, and since it took a long time for me to become mobile after my first birth, I figured I would need him for the whole two weeks to help my daughter get used to a less active mom and a new baby.

All through the pregnancy, I had worried that no one would get there in time for my labour. My first daughter came on a Sunday, preceded by lots of confusing sick feelings and then pain that had no traceable pattern or origin. By the time I admitted I was in labour, I was nearing transition and the midwives came to tell me that it was O.K. to push. I had had visions of the same relatively short and unrecognizable experience, and had worried that my three-year-old would be my only assistant at her sibling's birth. Now, I was sending my husband off to work. It seems the most consistent element of my birth experiences is denial.

My father also came once a week to take my daughter to the park, and today was his day. When he showed up a couple of hours later, I told him I might be in labour and that I might send for them at the park. Jordan and I intended to have our daughter at the birth. My mother, who was at work an hour away, had been given the job of looking after Evie during the labour and bringing her in when the baby was coming.

I called my student midwife, who asked about the pattern and frequency of my contractions. She said though I was probably in labour, I still sounded pretty happy. "Call me when it's not fun any more," she said. That made sense to me. I phoned my husband and told him to work through lunch, explaining that this was probably it, but not for a while. I called my mother to say the same. I called my friend in the neighbourhood and she was thrilled. I decided, as a novel experience, I would try to time the contractions. I hadn't had a chance to do it for my first baby, so I would try it for this one. I wrote about seven down but hadn't really got the hang of it by the time I had to get up and walk around. This isn't fun, I thought. I called the student midwife again. She agreed that she would start to get the midwives and their things together. My primary midwife had been called away because of a death in the family, but having become acquainted with most of the midwives through my three pregnancies, I was confident that I would feel good with whoever showed up. I also had complete confidence in the midwifery student. I knew my baby and I would literally be in good hands.

I now felt a change in myself and my labour that was quite pronounced, and I no longer wanted to be alone. But I had told my husband and my mother that they didn't need to hurry. Jordan was 45 minutes away and my mother an hour away. I didn't know if I could wait that long! I called my husband's office: "He's already gone. He knew you were farther along than you thought." I called my mother's work and someone said, "She left right after she got off the phone with you." I called my friend, who then packed her own new baby into the van and went over to the park to pick up my dad and my three-year-old.

My mother arrived first. Then my dad and Evie. I really wanted Evie to see me while I could still talk and not just concentrate on the labour. We had had several conversations about what labour and birth would be like, and we had watched a lot of videos. In fact, Jordan said she would soon be explaining birth to strangers on the bus. Even though we were well-prepared, I wanted to remind her that I would be making a lot of noises and that this would be really hard work, but that it was going to be a happy time. She looked at me, walked across the room, picked up her baby doll and brought it to me. "Mommy," she said, "I want to help you have the baby."

Jordan arrived and got me into a warm bath. The student midwife and my "second" midwife arrived. There was an initial bit of confusion while my mom tried to find ways to distract Evie, but then they were off amusing each other. I felt very glad to have my mother there so that I only had to concentrate on the labour. My mother kept Evie happy downstairs, while I laboured in my attic room with candles that the midwives would blow out whenever I left the room because it was so incredibly hot. I stayed very quiet in labour, knowing that if I lost my focus, I would become frightened and lose my ability to work through the contractions. I swayed back and forth between Jordan and the midwifery student, silently repeating to the baby: "This is your dad. This is the person who will catch you." When the midwifery student inched over to reach for something just a tiny way away, I started shaking my head and calling out. Even though no one was touching me, I needed to feel their physical presence right beside me. I had a sense that there were things going on outside my perception. But apart from the very annoying ring of the phone, they were peaceful things. I could hear the summer noises on the street. I could hear my dad and my daughter on the balcony one storey below the bedroom. A bit later I smelled something baking. They were all reassuring sensations that made me feel good in my space.

Then transition hit. The reason I knew it was transition was that this was when I began to feel like I was losing it. The midwifery student quietly suggested to Jordan that they unplug the phone, which was ringing off the hook. Jordan agreed and I started to cry and yell. I couldn't believe they would do something so inconsiderate! They left the phone where it was, promising not to touch it again. I also began saying, "I can't do it! I don't want to do it!" I believe I even said, "This isn't fun any more!" The other midwife had arrived by then, and she calmly asked what it was I couldn't do and didn't want to do. Did I want to change position? No, I just didn't want to have the baby! I wanted it to be over. Then both veteran midwives told me gently, sensibly and firmly that I would have to have the baby, and that was the only way it would be over. Of course, they also repeatedly told me how well I was doing. But what I heard was, my work was almost finished!

Pushing began and everything seemed fine. After transition, pushing comes as such a huge relief. The pushing urge was so strong I could do nothing but give in to it. I asked the midwives to bring in my little girl, who had been waiting downstairs with my mother. She came in, in between pushes, and she looked a little scared in my mom's arms. I said hi to her and she said hi to me. Then we talked about how mommy was going to be "loud loud" again and roar like a lion. She held on pretty tight to my mom, but she watched closely.

During my first birth, in between pushes, I had everyone guess whether I was having a girl or a boy. For my second, I focused on my kid in the breaks. The baby was crowning, and they asked me if I wanted to touch the head. I had no interest. There was a mirror I could have used to watch the head emerge. I didn't want it. As I had with Evie, I just concentrated on getting the baby out. And out the baby came in just a few pushes, and up onto my tummy. The cord was pretty short, so she couldn't come up high. Just as I had been with Evie, I felt totally wobbly after I had the baby and couldn't hold onto her slippery body. Jordan balanced the baby on my tummy. Then he and Evie cut the cord together.

I felt elated at having finished and began yelling, "That's it! I did it! I am done. I'm DONE!" while everyone else laughed at me and admired the baby. Evie was supposed to announce the baby's sex, but Jordan whispered first: "It's a girl!" Then we got Evie to look and she said, "It's a sister. I really wanted a sister." It was lovely, because throughout the pregnancy, I had been convinced I was having a boy and the only person who felt absolutely certain it was a girl was Evie. We called her Beatrice, which had been the only name that Evie, Jordan and I could agree on. Both of the children were born during June heat waves, in the same hour of the afternoon, in the same room.

To my surprise, my dad appeared around the corner of the door. He is notoriously squeamish. I was amazed that he was curious enough to come in, despite the fact that the room and I weren't cleaned up yet. An hour before, Jordan had invited him to stay, but he had been contemplating going home, thinking this could last all night. One of the midwives had informed him that this baby would arrive very soon.

I got cleaned up and we took pictures—another advantage of being prepared. After snuggling and kissing and stroking her sister, Evie told me they had been making a cake. They were intending to ice it, but it hadn't even had time to cool yet. She and my mom went to check on it.

I talked to the midwives about the labour and birth. I looked at the student midwife and said, "What was all that with the phone?" We were both baffled and laughing about my extreme reaction.

After the midwives tidied and left me and Jordan alone, Evie and my mom and dad came back with an iced green birthday cake, which we all ate together.

—*Miranda, mother of two*

## Cameras at the Birth

Opportunities to preserve your baby's birth on film abound. Some people choose a family member to photograph or videotape the baby's arrival; others hire a professional photographer or videographer; there are even television programs that regularly document the birth process.

If you choose to get your birth on film, make sure you don't assign the job to the very person you need at your side. It is probably better for your partner to be holding your hand than to remain hidden behind a camera while your baby emerges. But if this is your partner's preferred job, then make sure there is another person you would welcome at your side while you're pushing your baby out. It is almost impossible to provide labour support and be the official photographer at the same time.

Whoever is taking the pictures, amateur or professional, should be aware enough of what will occur and how to do the job that he or she stays well in the background. Any restrictions you may want to apply about pictures of your vagina should be well stated ahead of time. The focus of the birth should not be diverted to the camera, but should remain on you and the baby.

## Other Means of Support

As any mother will tell you, despite the importance of the birth experience, it's only the beginning. You will certainly have strong feelings about who should be there at this momentous time. But your need for others' support was probably evident much earlier in your pregnancy and will certainly be clear after the baby's birth. If there are people who cannot or should not attend the birth itself, you can still make use of their enthusiasm and abilities in other ways. For example, they could prepare meals ahead of time, phone friends and family to announce the birth, or spell off your partner in your first days after the big event.

## ◎ If You Want to Read More . . .

*The Birth Partner*, by Penny Simkin (Boston: The Harvard Common Press, 1989).

*Birthing From Within: An Extra-Ordinary Guide to Childbirth Preparation*, by Pam England and Rob Horowitz (Albuquerque, New Mexico: Partera Press, 1998).

*A Husband-Coached Childbirth*, by Robert A. Bradley (Sherman Oaks, California: Bantam, 1996).

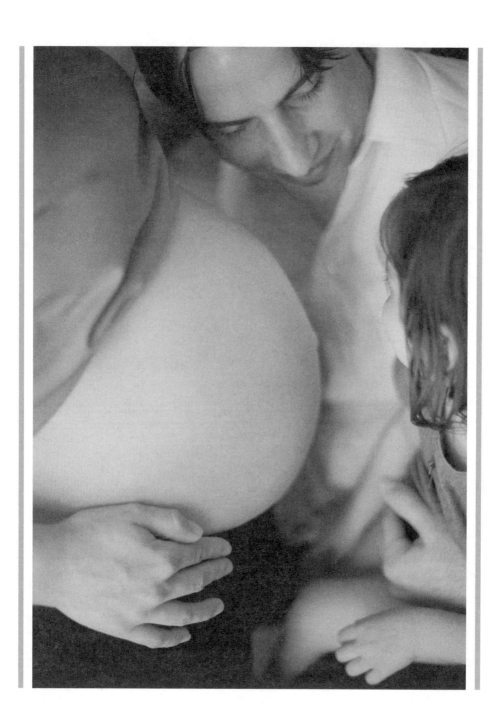

## Nine

◎ **The Last Few Weeks**

For many women, the last few weeks of pregnancy are emotionally charged. Knowing that most babies are born within 10 days of their due dates (that is, either 10 days before or after this date) gives them a sense that the birth could happen "any day now." Yet accumulation of discomforts stemming from their size and the baby's can make it feel like that baby will never come out!

If you feel anxious about the birth itself or wonder how you will cope with a new baby, then these feelings will also factor into your ability to rest and prepare yourself for what's ahead.

Most women visit their midwives on a weekly basis in the final month of their pregnancies. Midwives will often plan to visit you in your home at least once before the baby comes. This visit usually takes place around week 36 of your pregnancy.

As usual the midwife will check your urine and the baby's growth and position in your uterus. She will monitor your blood pressure particularly closely in the last few weeks and note any edema (swelling) in your hands or feet. You might be considering the test for the presence of group B streptococcus in your vagina at this stage so that decisions can be made regarding the use of antibiotics during labour. Sometimes, as the final week or two approaches, your midwife will discuss the option of an internal check to assess the ripeness of your cervix, which may help her judge your readiness to dilate when the moment arrives.

The midwives will probably repeatedly caution you to get rest. This may be difficult, especially now that you are large and may not be sleeping well. Like everything else, labour will seem more manageable when your energy is at its peak, and to get it there, you will need to sleep when you can.

Staying active is also important. Your midwives will speak to you about continuing to do exercise that you enjoy. Activities such as walking or swimming can help keep you healthy.

Talking about how to cope with the discomforts of pregnancy and your expectations of birth and new parenthood can also be important—now more than ever in the past nine months. Your midwife will probably discuss the signs and symptoms of labour and suggest when you should page her. Going over the plans that you have made will help to expose any lingering questions you may have. In these last weeks it is also important to review the way your midwife's practice covers midwives' days off, conditions for transfer and what you can expect if things don't go as planned.

## Preparing for Labour and Birth

Though you have probably already discussed the plans for your birth in detail, many more things may come up as the labour approaches. Your midwives can help you deal with these concerns and visualize how your labour may go.

What is it like to have a baby? Ask a dozen different women this question and you'll get a dozen different answers. Sure, there'll be some similarities, but the birth experience is as particular as it is universal. Women who tell their stories to other mothers at postpartum gatherings will hear similar stories, but they will also encounter birth experiences completely unlike their own.

Before Miranda had her first daughter, she was eager to have "the birth experience." Only afterward did she realize she hadn't had "the experience" at all but an experience particular to her circumstances, conditions and baby.

Though it is impossible to know what your labour and birth will be like, that doesn't mean that planning for the event is unwarranted. Most midwifery clients have a vision of the birth they want, which may actually have been what led them to midwifery in the first place.

### Making Plans

One of the popular concepts in many birth books these days is the *birth plan*. This is a document in which the mother describes her wishes for the birth, including everything from the environment she wants to create in the birth room to her feelings about the use of interventions.

Do you need a birth plan? That depends who you consider the birth plan to be for. Many advocates of birth plans assume the women writing them will encounter a medical staff person that may have a fairly routine way of dealing with labour, birth and the newborn. In this case, the birth plan is supposed to make the care the mother receives more personal. It is supposed to set the tone for the experience, even if the mother herself cannot articulate her needs because she is too far into labour.

But if you have midwives, you will be attended in labour and birth by people with whom you already have a relationship. In fact, your relationship will grow as you explore your feelings about pregnancy, birth and motherhood. Though midwives see birth as a normal occurrence, they do not consider it "routine." Even in the event of a transfer of care, the midwives will most likely be there to guide you through the more impersonal medical system.

So, if making your wishes known to an unfamiliar staff person is the only purpose of a birth plan, then you should not need to use one when in the care of your midwife.

On the other hand, sometimes the very act of writing about your birth can propel you to think about things in a new way and address the idea of birth. For people who fear birth, trying to imagine or articulate the experience of labour, birthing their baby and their first moments as parents can be a very useful exercise.

Some midwives suggest their clients write a birth story instead of a birth plan. The birth story includes all the elements that you might have touched upon in your birth plan, but it allows you to envision the event as an accomplishment, rather than as a future hurdle.

**Envisioning birth before labour starts**

I was still very nervous about how the pain was going to be and the fact that I had taken away the option of medication for pain relief by having my birth at home. Every time I had a doubt, though, the midwives assured me my body would know what to do. They asked me to write up a birth story describing how I imagined things would go. For the most part I believed it would all take place in my bathroom. In my birth story, I didn't feel the need to describe the things I would do. I saw it all as a journey from one state to another, with the final product being a baby. My birth didn't turn out a whole lot like what I had imagined, but it was relatively free of pain and uncomplicated. That was the journey I could only dream of and was blessed to have experienced.

—*Brandie, mother of one*

Whether you are writing a formal birth plan, envisioning a birth story or simply contemplating what you will need in labour, considering your birth experience ahead of time can help you address fears or concerns, solidify what you expect from yourself and your partner, and give you the impetus to gather whatever physical supplies you want to have on hand.

Going over your plan with your midwives and your personal support people can help you identify your expectations. The midwife may be able to point out things that need to be done. For example, if you want certain music playing, who will be in charge of making that happen? If you want a video of your birth, who will shoot it? They can help you pinpoint your needs and sort through what is of primary importance to you.

### Preparing for the Next Stages

As you near the end of your pregnancy, the time it takes to determine that you and the baby are still healthy is relatively short, but there is still a lot to fill an appointment with the midwife.

Now is when you should make sure your plans for recovery are in place.

Your midwives will probably talk to you about a strategy for caring for yourself after the baby comes. When you have already been up for the better part of 24 hours with a new baby, you will not have the energy to think about reinforcements. The midwives can help you form a realistic picture of postpartum life and help you think ahead about what you might need.

Although we give a lot of attention to preparing today's partners for labour and birth, we often don't talk enough about the importance of a woman's support people after birth. With their approach to birth as a life experience, rather than a medical event, midwives can help smooth the transition for you and your circle. Your baby will need to eat, sleep and be comforted after the birth, but so will you. Who will care for you while you look after your new son or daughter? Who will help you remember that you also need attention? In the last few appointments of prenatal care, the midwives can help you and your support people build a plan that will make your time with a newborn go as smoothly as possible.

## Gathering Supplies

Whether you plan to have your baby at home or at a hospital or birth centre, a good part of your labour usually takes place at home. This is especially true if you have a long early labour. You will want to make sure you have the supplies to make your chosen birth place comfortable for you, your support people and your baby. Your midwives will probably give you a specific list of supplies, suited to their practice. Birth supplies should be ready by 37 weeks. You can store them in a box or basket in the labour room.

*Supplies for Homebirth\**

- Disposable bed pads (36)
- Pillows (approximately 5)
- Washcloths (6)
- Receiving blankets (8 to 12)

\* This list and the next two should be used as a guideline. Discuss variations with your midwife.

- Newborn baby hat
- Clean linen: 2 fitted sheets, 2 flat sheets, pillowcases, towels (at least 3)
- Large plastic sheet for bed
- Safety pins
- 2 basins or pails
- Package of 10-cm x 10-cm sterile gauze pads (2 dozen)
- Hot water bottle
- Ice chips
- 2 small bags of frozen peas
- Small bottle of unopened olive oil
- Digital watch or a watch that has a second hand
- Food and drinks for mother, helpers and midwives
- Honey
- Gatorade or energy drink
- Gravol (oral or suppositories)
- 2 large garbage bags (one for dirty linen, one for garbage)
- Hand mirror
- Small bright lamp
- 2 extension cords
- Portable space heater
- Laundry detergent and stain remover
- 2 large cookie sheets or trays

*Supplies for Hospital or Birth Centre Birth*

To labour at home you need:
- Disposable bed pads (12)
- Pillows (approximately 5)
- 2 washcloths
- 2 basins or pails
- Food and drink for mother, helpers and midwives
- Honey
- Gatorade or energy drink

- Gravol (oral or suppositories)
- Hot water bottle
- Digital watch or a watch that has a second hand

Bring to the hospital or birth centre:
- 2 Pillows
- Basin or bag for the car
- Blanket (for car)
- Food
- Small bottle of unopened olive oil
- Hand mirror
- Small change for phone, vending machines, etc.
- Overnight bag (including slippers)
- Infant car seat
- Baby clothes (including baby hat)
- Newborn diapers

*Postpartum supplies (for home, birth centre or hospital)*
- A large package of menstrual pads
- Squeeze bottle (such as a small empty dish-soap bottle)
- Extra-strength Tylenol (optional)
- Natural oil for baby skin (almond, olive)
- Calendula or zinc cream
- Digital thermometer (with Celsius reading)
- Lots of diapers, receiving blankets, undershirts and sleepers or nighties
- Breast pump (optional)

The lists provided here might seem long, but most items are easy to find and they will be useful when the time comes. Newborn diapers and gauze pads sound like things you should have at a birth, but right now, you probably cannot fathom why you need honey, olive oil or frozen peas.

*Grocery and Household Items*

These items serve various purposes at a birth. Honey is an excellent source of energy, and taking a spoonful when your strength and enthusiasm are waning may give you the boost that will help you go on. Olive oil is used for massaging the perineum and helping the skin to stretch without tearing when the baby is making his or her exit. Frozen peas provide an excellent compress for a swollen pelvic floor after the birth. Unlike an ice pack, they mould well to your body.

Cookie sheets can be used in two ways at a birth. One cookie sheet can serve as a surface on which midwives can place their instruments. A cookie sheet with a heating pad on top can be used to heat receiving blankets and act as a warming bed if your baby needs it. Gravol may help you sleep.

*Preparing Your Space*

Wash and rinse all the sheets in hot water, dry them on a hot setting, then store them in plastic bags sealed with tape, or put them in bins with lids. When it is time to make up the birth bed, put a fitted sheet and a flat sheet on the bed as you normally would. Then put a plastic sheet over these. (You can use a fitted plastic sheet or a shower curtain, pinned at the corners.) Make up the bed a second time over top. After you have the baby, your helpers can simply strip the bed and you will have a fresh bed made underneath.

*As You Labour*

Having food on hand for a labour and birth at home is important, as you don't want your support people dashing out to the grocery store. You may also want to plan to bring food to the hospital not only for you but for your support people and your midwives too. It will mean that they don't have to rely on vending machines and cafeterias.

You should have two basins or pails for preparing compresses. You will also need these in case you throw up.

Many people like to keep the lights dimmed in the birthing room, but the midwives may need a clear view as your baby begins to crown or for suturing after the birth. Rather than turning on all the lights, they can use the small lamp, attached to an extension cord, to focus the light where they need it.

A hand mirror will give you the option of seeing your baby's head emerge.

*After the Birth*

You will need menstrual pads for after the birth. Paper or cotton pads are preferable because pads with plastic or a "dry weave" can slow healing.

Your perineum may feel quite tender after you have pushed your baby out. Filling a squeeze bottle with warm water and rinsing the vaginal area during urination can be very soothing.

A breast pump is something you may never require; but if you do need one you could find yourself without this vital piece of equipment at 3:00 A.M. on a Sunday. Though there are many such devices on the market, finding one that will work for you is not as easy as grabbing the first one you find on the drugstore shelf. If you buy a breast pump, be sure to research the possibilities—both by talking to other moms and by reading up on the different kinds. Borrowing a breast pump or two for the first couple of weeks of nursing can be a great way to see what model you prefer.

## Planning for Times when Things Don't Go as Planned

No birth will happen exactly the way you expect it to.

Acknowledging this fact does not mean that you are setting yourself up for disaster. It just means you can make provisions in case your plans or needs change. Planning ahead can make it more likely your birth will be the way you want, even if it's not the way you planned.

**Valuable research**

We were made aware of what the protocols would be under various circumstances. But we should have taken advantage of our midwife's offer to meet two of her clients who had already become parents with her help. We definitely should have taken the hospital tour as well. When we did have our baby, and we did have to transfer to the hospital, I was left feeling confused and uncertain about what awaited us there.

—*Mike, father of one*

Taking some basic precautions is a good thing to do. Say, for example, your mother is supposed to be coming from Florida to look after your first child. Why not have a backup person in place in case you go into labour early? You are planning a homebirth? It's probably a good idea to pre-register at a local hospital. If you decide to go in for some extra assistance, then your support people can stay with you instead of going through reams of paperwork.

## Waiting

A lot of labour preparation simply involves waiting. Sometimes this can seem like the most difficult aspect of all. The constant state of readiness itself can be exhausting.

It may seem impossible, but now is the time to savour your relative freedom, if you can. If you have other children, try to arrange some events at which you can give them special attention without having to factor in a nursing infant. If you do make such plans, you may want to announce them on a daily basis rather than too far ahead, in order to avoid disappointing your older children if the birth forces a cancellation. Now can also be a good time to enjoy your relationship with your partner, go out with friends or do things completely on your own.

Because babies do have their own schedules, it's a good idea to make any plans for birth or aftercare somewhat fluid. We have heard dozens of stories of people booking time off work to help out a new mom or attend a birth, only to find that the baby's schedule doesn't accommodate the appointment book. Or of people who were supposed to move residences right before a baby came, and who ended up with a car seat in the moving van. If you can, try not to make your deadlines too tight.

## Overdue

"Don't worry, it has to come out eventually." Pregnant women everywhere have comforted themselves with this mantra. Miranda repeated it nightly while waiting for her second child. But how long past the calculated due date is too long for the baby to stay *in utero*?

Opinions on this vary, even among midwives. Traditionally, midwives were more likely to let a pregnancy progress past the due date, and doctors tended to intervene by inducing labour. Different provinces have different regulations about when midwives need to consult with a physician about a post-term pregnancy. What remains consistent is the midwives' commitment to helping you make informed decisions regarding monitoring your later-than-expected arrival. Should induction be warranted, they will offer you some techniques for encouraging your baby that don't necessitate a hospital stay.

Passing your due date can be very frustrating. If you are overdue, you will probably feel anxious for labour to start. What caregivers need to determine is whether your baby is also eager to arrive. If you are experiencing a lack of movement, or if you are overdue, your midwives may talk to you about testing the fluctuations of your baby's heart rate or assessing his or her movements, breathing and the amniotic fluid for signs of stress. If you decide to go ahead with these tests and they indicate that the baby is no longer thriving, a physician will induce labour or schedule a C-section. One way of determining your baby's continuing health *in utero* is to check on his or her environment and responses to certain stimuli.

### Non-stress Tests

One mother we know who had a few occasions to have a non-stress test for her baby wryly said that the baby's stress level was probably fine; it was hers she worried about. This type of test is done with two ultrasound monitors, one to measure your contractions and one to measure the baby's heart rate. The monitors are attached to a larger machine that spits out a paper strip containing the information your caregivers need to assess your baby. They are looking for the kinds of accelerations that are normal as the baby moves around. The test usually takes from 20 to 60 minutes.

If the result is normal, you will probably just sign up to come back for the same test in a few days. This is a way to monitor your baby's health. If the result raises questions, then you will probably be scheduled for a biophysical profile.

### Biophysical Profiles

A more involved test that uses ultrasound is the biophysical profile (BPP). The BPP measures four factors: the baby's body movements, breathing movements and muscle tone, and the amount of amniotic fluid in the sac around the baby. The latter will be examined very carefully since it is a significant sign of fetal well-being. If your test indicates that the baby is not doing well, an induction will be planned immediately.

Sometimes only the non-stress test and the measure of amniotic fluid are necessary. These two indicators can often give your practitioner sufficient information to assess of your baby's health.

None of these tests is more invasive than an ultrasound, but they may be tedious. The results can help in making decisions about what, if any, kind of induction to pursue. If your overdue time stretches out, the tests may have to be repeated every three to four days, or more often.

### Home Inductions

Everything from rides on a bumpy road to pizza with hot peppers has been given credit for starting labour. It is hard to know what really works, but many of the non-medical methods of labour induction that were popular generations ago are still used today.

Although it might be difficult for some overdue women to contemplate increasing physical activity, it may jostle that baby into some extra activity too. You could try walking stairs or aggressive vacuuming, but it's important not to overexert yourself to the point that, when labour begins, you're too tired out to work through it.

Nipple stimulation can cause the uterus to contract. You can do this by yourself or with your partner's help. This activity, which may sound enjoyable in other circumstances, can be a chore when you are trying to bring on labour. While it seems straightforward, it actually requires time and effort: it needs to be done several times a day for 15 minutes at a time. Consult your midwife before trying this.

Sexual activity has also been known to encourage labour. This works for some women partially because sexual arousal releases oxytocin. Seminal fluid contains a natural prostaglandin. Both substances cause the uterus to contract. The same hormones are sometimes used in hospital inductions.

Other home remedies for an overdue baby include taking evening primrose oil, either orally or as a vaginal suppository, drinking tea made of blue or black cohosh, and ingesting castor oil. If you are interested in herbal inductions, discuss this with your midwife. She may be able to advise you about the frequency and size of the doses, and will remain on standby in case they have the desired effect. Alternatively, she may refer you to a skilled naturopath or herbalist. There are also several herbal books that include instructions about dosages (see the If You Want to Read More . . . section at the end of this chapter for suggestions). It is important to acknowledge that there is a lack of scientific research about herbs and that the label "natural" is often mistaken for "harmless."

Castor oil, in particular, requires a special caution. You may take several doses of evening primrose oil without noticing any effect. Although castor oil may or may not get labour started, it will affect you. It will probably purge your system, giving you diarrhea and perhaps making you temporarily unable to hold down food. It might also bring your labour on in a very effective and rapid manner. Always consult your midwife if you are about to try a home remedy to induce labour.

## Midwife Assists

*Stretch and Sweep*

Sometimes a midwife will try to encourage the cervix to open slightly by gently stretching it and sweeping her finger around the inside. The procedure, which may result in some discomfort and bleeding, can cause the release of the hormone prostaglandin and sometimes "jump-starts" labour.

*Rupturing Membranes*

Under specific circumstances (for example, if your cervix is fully ripe or you are trying to avoid chemical inductions), your midwife may try to help labour along by breaking the sac of membranes holding your baby and the amniotic fluid. This procedure is performed with a very small hook inserted through the cervix. The membranes break, "waters" flow out and the baby's head then presses against the cervix, opening it so that labour begins or proceeds more efficiently. Though this procedure is no more uncomfortable than a vaginal exam, it is still an intervention and needs to be monitored closely.

## Hospital Inductions

If your baby needs to come out, and you have forgone or not succeeded with home inductions, then you will probably proceed to the hospital for medical induction of labour.

At the hospital, one of two procedures may be used to bring on labour, or both may be applied in combination. Prostaglandin gel is a topical application for softening the cervix, which makes it easier for the cervix to open and the baby to pass through. The gel may be applied once or several times over a period of hours or even a couple of days. Sometimes the gel is applied at the hospital and then the woman may go home to wait for labour to start.

Oxytocin (also called Pitocin), a labour-inducing drug that is given to the mother in an intravenous drip, causes uterine contractions. To receive this treatment, you must remain in hospital so your response to the drug can be monitored, and the dosage adjusted to get labour started and keep it going. If a hospital induction is required, your midwife can remain with you, although her role may be altered. For example, she may transfer your care to a medical team and continue as labour support or assist the doctors with their work.

Some women are more than ready to have their baby by the ninth month. Others feel their babies arrive before they feel fully prepared. Sometimes it seems that women who want more time have babies who are eager to arrive, while impatient women have children who are less likely to show up on time!

## ◈ If You Want to Read More . . .

*Birthing From Within: An Extra-Ordinary Guide to Childbirth Preparation*, by Pam England and Rob Horowitz (Albuquerque, New Mexico: Partera Press, 1998).

*The Complete Book of Pregnancy and Childbirth* (new ed.), by Sheila Kitzinger (London: Dorling Kindersley Limited, 1996).

*Healthy Beginnings: Your Handbook for Pregnancy and Birth* (2nd ed.), by The Society of Obstetricians and Gynecologists of Canada (Ottawa: The Society of Obstetricians and Gynecologists of Canada, 2000).

*Pregnancy and Birth: The Best Evidence*, by Joyce Barrett and Teresa Pitman (Toronto: Key Porter Books, 1999).

*The Mother of All Pregnancy Books: An All-Canadian Guide to Conception, Birth & Everything in Between*, by Ann Douglas (Toronto: CDG Books, 2000).

*Wise Woman Herbal for the Childbearing Year*, by Susun S. Weed (Woodstock, New York: Ash Tree Publishing, 1986).

*Your Pregnancy Week-by-Week*, by Glade B. Curtis (Tucson, Arizona: Fisher Books, 1994).

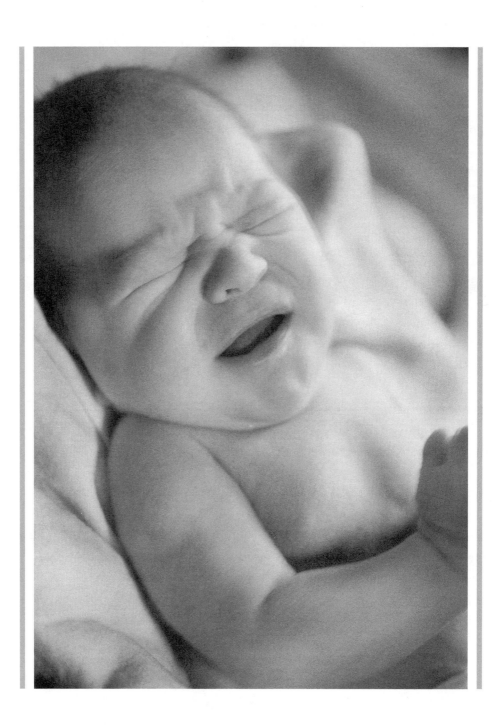

## Ten

### The Birth Experience

### Getting Started

When is it really labour? Good question. The flip answer is that you'll know when it's really labour. Eventually this is true, because you'll have a baby in your lap. But you may well be in the early stages of labour without realizing it.

Even the definition of "real" versus "false" labour is debatable. Though you may have been having "Braxton Hicks" contractions (a tightening of the belly that may occur on and off for several weeks or months before birth), your labour may be real. The uterus gets good practice doing this work, and tightenings in your cervix in the final few days or weeks of pregnancy could be the beginning of effective ripening that will help when labour becomes active.

If life were a sitcom, we would all make great splashes on the grocery store floor as our water broke, or heavy contractions would begin in an elevator. In real life, signs of early labour are rarely so definitive.

#### Breaking Waters

When women refer to their water breaking, they are talking about what happens when the sac that the baby is in breaks and the amniotic fluid leaks out. Fewer than 20 percent of labours begin with the water breaking, and a significant number of these labours are not followed immediately by contractions.

Your water can break in a big gush, but a tiny trickle is no less significant. Many women who have a smaller leak confuse it with urinary incontinence—a not uncommon occurrence in later pregnancy. If you are not sure which you are having, use a menstrual pad and note the flow, colour and so on. Amniotic fluid is clear and smells different from urine. Fluid may leak continuously, or in small gushes, as you and your baby move around. If you aren't sure whether your water has broken, your midwives can use a little paper test strip that will show if amniotic fluid is present.

Though many labours that begin with the water breaking do not get going right away, your caregivers will want to keep track of the length of time between the water breaking and the start of active labour. It used to be standard practice for doctors to induce labour if a woman was not having strong contractions within 24 hours of her water breaking. Midwives, and many doctors, now see this intense countdown as unnecessary. However, because the amniotic fluid acts as a barrier around your baby, protecting him or her from infection, there are certain things that you should not do after your water has broken. Your midwives will guide you through any changes you need to make in normal activity until labour begins.

### Mucous Plug or "Bloody Show"

Losing your mucous plug, or "having a bloody show," may be another indicator that the baby is on the way. The mucous plug is a cap at the opening of the cervix that is released when the cervix starts to dilate. When this happens some people notice a streak of yellow or pink when they go to the washroom, as the plug disintegrates. Sometimes the entire plug pops out at once.

A "bloody show" is a *small* amount of darker pink or red blood, usually noticed when wiping after going to the bathroom. (Too much red bleeding can be a sign of a problem and should be reported immediately to your midwife.)

Labour can start anytime from a few minutes after you lose your plug to a few days later, and some women never actually see the plug in its whole or disintegrated form, because they are too far into labour when it is released.

### Discomforts and Mood

Some women feel as if they are getting their periods before labour begins. They may get cramps or their stomachs may get very upset.

Others report significant changes in mood. Sometimes people who felt anxious and dreaded the prospect of another day of pregnancy say they woke up one day feeling like they were no longer cranky about being big and uncomfortable. That was the day labour began.

There is, of course, the infamous "nesting urge," which drives people to clean obsessively or otherwise prepare their home for the baby. Though mothers near their due date should probably be relaxing, many of us engage in some sort of preparation, so it's hard to tell the practical urge from the instinctive. Needless to say, while the nesting urge definitely strikes some people very hard, it is not a definite indicator of labour.

### Contractions

Many women's bodies skip any other indicators of labour and go straight to contractions. The majority of labours will have recognizable contractions at some point, though at first the contractions may be mild and hard to detect. One of the best descriptions of contractions likens them to a belt tightening and releasing. You may feel them in your belly or your lower back.

Contractions early in labour are often all over the place—long, then short, a few minutes apart, and then half an hour apart. How far along you are in labour is often determined by the length of each contraction and how far apart contractions are from one another. Most labours will settle into a definite pattern as they progress, and you—or your personal support people—will be able to keep track of this pattern and pass the information along to your midwife before she arrives. However, in the early stages of many labours, the pattern of contractions is usually completely erratic until the body settles into a rhythm.

Infrequently, the contractions do not take on a noticeable rhythm; rather, they fluctuate wildly while still remaining frequent and intense, until near transition.

Some midwives recommend that if you are really unsure about whether you are in labour, you should take a bath (provided your waters haven't broken yet). Your labour may either peter out or intensify in the water, or when you step out of the tub.

You could also try lying down to get some rest. Whether or not you are in labour today, the rest will be good for you, and if you manage to sleep through part of your labour, all the better.

You may want to try timing a few contractions to see if they are coming regularly and how long they last. You don't need to time every single contraction, just a few at a time, every so often. Consider this a diagnostic tool, not a method of controlling your labour. Watching the clock can make your progress seem unbelievably slow.

*Timing Your Contractions*

Make sure you use a digital watch or one with a second hand. Start timing at the beginning of the contraction and note the time. Register when the contraction finishes as well. The difference between the two is the length (duration) of your contraction. To figure out how frequently you are having contractions, calculate the time elapsed from the start of one to the start of the next. You might be in early labour when the contractions are regular and about 15 to 45 seconds long and anywhere from five to twenty minutes apart. Labour is considered to be active when the contractions are 45 to 60 seconds long and three to five minutes apart consistently.

## A sample contraction chart

| Start | Finish | Length of contraction | How far apart |
|-------|--------|----------------------|---------------|
| 12:01:30 | 12:02:10 | 40 seconds | 3 minutes 40 seconds |
| 12:05:10 | 12:06 | 50 seconds | 3 minutes 20 seconds |
| 12:08:30 | 12:09:12 | 42 seconds | [etc.] |

## When to Call Your Midwife

If you have any genuine indicators that labour is going to start, call your midwife to alert her. It will probably be very exciting for you to realize that the pregnancy will be coming to an end in a matter of hours or days; however, unless you are in active labour, this exchange of information can take place during daytime hours. If you start having contractions at suppertime, by all means give your midwife a call. She will appreciate knowing that you may need her in the middle of the night. If you start having contractions at 3:00 A.M., it is better to let your midwives get some rest until breakfast time so that they can be in good shape for the hours of more active labour ahead. Of course, if there are any signs that labour is progressing suddenly and rapidly, then you should call regardless of the time.

## Birth Preparations

Early labour, when you are unsure whether you are really in labour at all, is a good time to go over your game plan with regard to birth preparations.

### Calling Support People

When you get your first indication that you may be in labour, you should alert your personal support people. This doesn't mean they have to rush home from work right away, but it gives everyone the opportunity to prepare and lends a less harried air to your baby's birth. Anyone who is playing a support role at the birth itself should be alerted, as should anyone who may be providing child or pet care, so that they can clear their schedule.

Thinking you are in labour may inspire a lot of phone calls, even to people who will not be present. It can be great to share the news. But though the baby's birth seems tantalizingly close now, it may still be many, many hours before he or she arrives. People who have been told that labour has begun often get anxious for regular updates. When your phone starts ringing off the hook while you try to stay focused during a contraction, you may curse yourself for having called everyone from Prince Edward Island to British Columbia. Try to anticipate the possible results of your labour announcement. If you do decide to make calls, request that your friends and family wait for further news from you before phoning, so that you can keep the line clear and labour without worrying about providing progress reports.

### *Locating and Arranging Supplies*

Though you may feel that laying out supplies for your home or hospital birth is a little premature if you have just had your first few mild contractions, remember: you will not be up for it later. Go over the supplies with your support people and remind anyone who is helping you where they can find things like drinks, towels, olive oil and clean washcloths. Make sure there is film in your camera! Do you have extra batteries on hand? You may also want to make up your birth bed now.

Make sure your hot water tank is turned up. This is essential if you'll be filling a birthing pool, but you will probably want to take showers or baths whether you plan to have your baby in your own bed or in hospital. No one need boil water unless your hot water tank is empty or you want tea.

## The Midwives' Arrival

Regardless of where you plan to have your baby, the midwives often come to your home to help you work through labour. Though they may come to check on your progress early in labour, their real role is during active labour when they can help you work through pain and encourage you through to the birth.

Most women can handle early labour on their own. This means that the midwives may pay a short visit to your home once or twice before settling in to stay. This can be discouraging, but it is part of their effort to help you pace yourself as you work to get your baby out. You may have had regular contractions for several hours, but if you are only slightly dilated and you can still talk and walk during contractions, then the midwives will usually leave you to rest. They will return when your labour becomes more active.

### Encouragement breeds confidence

With my second birth, when my midwife checked my dilation, she didn't have to tell me how many centimetres I was dilated; she just said, "Wow, you've done a great job already. You're amazing." And I was.

With my first birth [with a doctor], my experience of being checked on was "We'll let you know when you are ready to have this baby—we're the authority." With my midwife, the most wonderful thing was that nobody ever told me what to do—ever. They just listened to me and talked to me. My body and I were in harmony and powerful together. I'll never forget being that powerful in all those elements of myself.

—*Ruth, mother of two*

When one of your midwives does come over and decides to stay, you can be sure that your baby really is on its way. Most often, the second midwife will arrive as you near transition or the pushing phase. For Miranda, just seeing the "backup" midwife come in made her realize that she could make it through to the end.

## Coping During Labour

When some women labour, they do it in a heightened state of awareness so that that touch on the back may feel too hard or too light; or they may want the lighting in the room to be adjusted, or the window to be opened or closed. Other women lose all awareness of what is going on around them and only focus on their bodies. Women occasionally enter an almost trancelike state and forget that they are in labour at all.

These are all very personal means of coping with the incredible task the body is doing, and they are quite unconscious for many people. But the midwives and your support people will be able to help you try other ways of finding comfort as you work on moving your baby through the birth canal.

### Working toward a "natural" birth

Exactly one week after my due date, while lying in bed, I felt wetness between my legs. Not the gush they warn you about but enough of a dribble to feel wet for the next hour. The next day I told the midwife what had happened, and she confirmed that my water had indeed broken, although likely only a little. Nonetheless, I was told that if labour didn't start within four days, I would have to go to the hospital to be induced. Which would mean giving up my plan for a homebirth. To encourage labour, I took homeopathic pills. By Friday morning it wasn't working and I felt desperate. The one thing I wanted more than anything was to at least try to have a homebirth.

The next step involved drinking that awful castor oil. My midwife explained the procedure carefully. When I told both my mother and my Jamaican boss about it, both said that women had been doing it for decades, back before hospital inductions took over. Around 1:00 P.M. on Friday I mixed up the castor oil with orange juice, and thought I'd make it taste better by adding chipped ice. When I tried to drink it, it got stuck in my throat so that I gagged and threw it all up. The second time I skipped the ice and it was much better. I took a second dose an hour later, then waited. This gave me much-appreciated time to reread all the notes and letters I'd received from women who had attended my special shower two weeks earlier.

By 5:00 P.M., things started rumbling and the castor oil began its infamous purging. I had diarrhea almost hourly for the next few hours, till I felt sure that I was "cleaned out." Still no contractions. Nonetheless, expecting the baby to arrive sometime soon, my partner and I made the plan to have my stepsons (ages six and nine at the time) sleep over at our house for that particular weekend. They had been part of the plan for the birth all along. Our midwives had loaned us home videos of other women's births to show them ahead of time. The boys were well prepared and had requested to be there for the event, so we had agreed.

Around 11:00 P.M., just as I was getting ready for bed, my water broke. This time I felt the pop and the gush. I knew for sure. So I showed my partner. We then cleaned it up and went to bed.

At 1:00 A.M., I woke up and felt my first contraction. Not painful, but significant enough to know it was the real thing. I started writing in my journal and timing the contractions. My partner slept beside me in bed, completely unaware of the movements. After two hours, I moved from the bed to the floor. I had thrown up several times and had difficulty drinking or eating anything. By 4:00 A.M., I was in the washroom, moving between taking showers and just sitting on the toilet waiting to throw up again. I don't think I spoke at all during this time or made any sounds. I just let my body go with the flow. Also, I deliberately didn't want to wake up my partner or call my midwife, because I wanted them to be fresh and rested when I needed them. And quite frankly, I enjoyed labouring on my own.

By 5:00 A.M. the contractions were getting harder and I decided to phone my midwife. Unfortunately, my independence ended up working against me: my primary midwife got a page for another birth five minutes before I called her, so she didn't get to come to my birth. Hearing me make the phone call, my partner woke up and sprang into action. He lined the bed with plastic, called my parents in Indiana and told them to start driving. Then he phoned his brother to come be with my stepsons. He was fresh, rested and ready for action, just as I'd hoped.

By the time the first midwife arrived at my house around 6:00 A.M., she checked me and I was already 10 centimetres dilated! She quickly paged for the second midwife. The contractions were hard by this time, but I had slipped into an altered state and could barely feel them, even though I had taken nothing for the pain. I also forgot to do some of the breathing and meditation exercises that I'd planned for myself. It seems I didn't need them. I was completely oblivious to the background music that I planned to have playing. (My partner insists that there was music playing, but that part's a blur.)

Since I was already completely dilated, my midwife asked me to push. But I had no desire to push; my contractions had almost stopped, so I went to sleep for an hour instead while we waited for the second midwife to arrive, thereby also giving them time to get set up and ready for the actual baby. When the second midwife arrived at around 7:00 A.M. I reluctantly woke up and started to walk around, at their suggestion. Within minutes the contractions returned.

The midwives gently suggested pushing positions for me to try, using my partner as a support. It was an incredibly unifying experience for us, which the midwives get credit for. At the pushing stage, we started taking photos. We have photos of each of the positions, and we both look so happy and confident. But the pushing was hard and painful and lasted nearly three hours. Though it was the hardest part so far, it certainly didn't feel as if it had taken that long.

Midway through the pushing stage, my stepsons woke up and came in to check on the progress. Although they were sleeping just in the next room, they had slept through most of the action, since it was so surprisingly quiet. Their uncle made them breakfast, and then everyone floated in and out of the birthing room at will. It worked out well to have someone there to take care of the kids' needs, so my partner could stay by my side at all times. The kids found it a bit boring because this part seemed to take so long, but when the baby's head started pushing out they came in the room and stayed until the actual birth.

So finally, after just a little more than nine hours from the first contraction, Adrian was born, at 10:23 A.M. He came out with a final tear and was caught by my partner. Immediately he started crying, which the midwives explained as "telling his birth story and how hard the last hours had been for him." Both stepsons got to hold their new brother while the umbilical cord was still attached. My partner cut the cord. The moment after the baby came out, I felt fabulous. All I knew was that the pain was over. It was even as if in that moment all memory of the pain disappeared.

For the first few hours after the birth we ate, rested and cleaned up. The bed was surprisingly neat, despite all the blood I lost, and nothing got stained. I was so relieved to just be home and to have my family and friends around me. The midwives taught me to breastfeed, and Adrian caught on almost immediately. Later in the day, my friend from the apartment upstairs came down with her three-month-old baby, and she, my mother and I all worked together to get Adrian to latch on again before bedtime that first day. It was much harder than the first time with the midwives, but we got the hang of it!

Having a baby has been a transformative experience for me. The birth was a powerful moment for me, my partner and our family. The choice to have a midwife be a part of this experience was an easy, obvious one for me. I was surprised at how strongly I felt about certain aspects of the birth and the amazing way that the midwives worked with me to achieve my dreams for my baby's entrance into the world. I am absolutely convinced that if I had not had midwives, I would not have had the natural, intervention-free birth and beginning that I was able to provide for my baby. I feel confident that my baby has had the best possible beginning to his wonderful life.

—*Linda, mother of one, stepmother of two*

### Sleep and Rest

Some people find it impossible to sleep and rest even in the earliest stages of labour, but these things are vital to keeping the labouring mother's energy up. So, at the first sign of labour the best thing to do may be to have a nap! Even if you can't drop off to sleep completely, lying down may help. Some women are even able to get a bit of sleep after labour is well established. The quiet time, with a silent companion or on their own, can be very calming, even though labour is intensifying.

*Food and Drinks*

For years the hospital standard was to keep women from eating or drinking during labour, in case a C-section was warranted. But if you think about the enormous physical exertion a woman goes through in labour, and compare it with running a marathon, you see how it may not make sense to expect the body to function well without calories and liquid.

This doesn't mean you will feel like eating a huge plate of curry when you are in labour. However, having some food that is easy to digest may be a good way to keep up your strength. Early in labour, take the opportunity to eat; as labour progresses, continue to eat small portions of healthy food if you can. Drinking is important throughout, whether you feel that you want to make the effort to drink or not. Dehydration is not good for you or the baby. Drinking liquids that the body can absorb quickly will benefit you. Electrolyte solutions, such as Gatorade, are a good thing to have on hand. You will probably not remember to drink them when you most need them, but your support people and your midwives can keep pressing them on you. You will thank them later.

*Distraction*

Since many first labours involve a long initial stage before contractions become really intense, it's good to have some distractions at hand. Some women like to spend the early stages of labour reminding themselves of how their lives are about to change; others find it helpful to distract themselves so that they don't watch the clock constantly. A stack of magazines or videos you have been saving can be a treat to crack open along with your birthing supplies.

*Water*

Whether or not you hope to have a water birth, using water while you labour can be a great coping mechanism. Standing in the shower or sitting in the tub while your midwives or personal support people pour water over your belly is a wonderful way to relax during the contractions. It can also help speed up a labour that is moving along but not yet active.

*Movement and Changes of Position*

Movement is one of the greatest coping tools that a labouring mother can employ. Climbing stairs, going back and forth to the bathroom, going outside and around the block if the weather is good can provide wonderful distractions. These activities also help the baby move more efficiently through the birth canal.

Changing positions in labour—from upright to sitting to squatting to lying down to rolling onto all fours—can help bring the baby down. In addition it helps move the pressure from within to different areas of your back, belly and pelvis so that nothing becomes a "hot spot" for too long. If a labour is progressing too slowly, the midwives will suggest positions that may speed the process up. If a baby is coming quickly, then the midwives can try to slow the baby by helping you move into another position.

It's possible for a mother to hold many positions on her own. But her partner or another support person can also be of great assistance in getting her into a squat or lean and helping her to hold these positions. Sitting on the toilet or crouching on a birthing ball or stool can be a good way to get into a position that might be difficult without assistance.

**Confidence at home with midwives**

As we had been with our past two babies, we were once again past that magic due date on the calendar, but our visits in the midwives' office were still upbeat. The midwives kept telling me that things were going to happen and not to be afraid. I believe that between my husband and me, we must have asked about 1,000 times when the midwives would come to the house, how long they would stay with us, when we might transfer to the hospital, when we should call, etc.

Labour began teasing me on Thursday evening, starting and stopping, and continued in this manner for two full days. Saturday I had itchy feet and needed to get out. So we loaded up our 3-year-old and our 16-month-old and went walking at a car show. Crazy, since it was −30° C! Labour finally began slowly during the night.

My midwife on call was fantastic. She reminded me not to watch the clock and to try to get some rest. I thought she was crazy since I was not in any mood to sleep! Around 8:00 A.M. I began my day by having a bath and generally feeling nervous and lost about the whole process. I called my midwife once more. She encouraged me to get up and keep moving around. By 11:00 A.M. the contractions started to feel stronger. We tried to walk outside, but every time I moved the contractions would come on top of each other. I was losing the good humour on which I pride myself. So at noon I requested that someone come over so that I could know if I was advancing or not. My midwives arrived to find me well into labour.

Like my other two babies, this one was also posterior (head down, but facing the wrong direction). But this time the position of my baby did not cause me to panic. I simply drew on the confidence of the midwives. They suggested that I begin to run up and down my basement stairs to help the baby turn. He turned in a matter of 25 minutes, and we went on to deliver in our own home an hour after that. Thank goodness we did not need to transfer to the hospital.

*—Joanne, mother of three*

*Touch*

Not all women want to be touched during labour. However, for those who appreciate encouraging physical contact from their support people, touch can be a very powerful tool for dealing with labour pain. The midwives will be able to show your partner or another support person how to apply counter pressure for back pain during labour. Massaging a labouring mother's feet, hands and shoulders can also provide great relief. A lighter technique than massage is effleurage. This involves using the flat of the hand or fingers to make long stroking movements on the thighs, back or belly, which can provide relief and relaxation.

*Sound*

Some women remain quiet during labour, some women are very loud, and many are a combination of the two. The third "type" may be quiet and "Zenlike" while working through contractions, but loud and ferocious while pushing. During labour, Sarah vocalized the word "open" as a deep drawn-out sound, and she visualized her cervix opening to allow her baby out. She is sure that this helped her stay focused.

If you are vocalizing during labour, the kind of sound that you make can actually help or hinder you. Strange but true! Bear with us: a high sound, such as a scream or a shriek, is the kind of sound we tend to make when we feel frightened and tense. A lower, more guttural sound, the kind you make while you are biking up a steep hill or heaving groceries, is a sound that works with your body's exertion. If you are making sounds, the midwives will help you try to keep your sound, and your body, open so that all the parts of you work in concert.

## A Planned Hospital or Birth Centre Birth— Making the Move

If you are planning a hospital birth, you and your midwives will have discussed at what point in your labour you will move to the hospital. Different midwives make different arrangements with their clients. The goal is generally to allow labour to progress as long as possible at home while getting to the hospital in plenty of time for the pushing stage and the baby's birth. The distance of your home from the hospital or birth centre will be a determining factor.

Familiarizing yourself with the route to the hospital that has the fewest potential obstacles is a good plan, as is making sure your car is clean and there is enough room for you to get into as comfortable a position as possible.

### Feeling at home in the hospital

I was expecting my first baby, and I wanted to be in a secure environment, mostly because I felt like I didn't know what would happen. I wasn't planning on having an epidural, but I wanted to be in an environment where that was a possibility. The hospital offered a combination of security, access to pain medication and convenience. It was also a neutral place for our families to visit us afterwards. They could come to see the baby. Then I could go home with my husband and my new baby and not have a lot of people coming into my space.

I was 10 days late, so after some discussion the midwives did a stretch and sweep on the Friday. I also had acupuncture and went to a homeopath. I wanted some action, so on Saturday I went for a three-hour walk. Sunday my water broke. The midwives came over to check me, but I wasn't really having contractions. So they went home and I went to bed. At about 3:00 A.M., I started having contractions, but they were totally manageable: about six minutes apart. The midwives came to check again, but we agreed that I didn't need them yet. So they went away again. I took some Gravol, hoping to get some sleep, but I wasn't able to.

They came back in the afternoon, but things didn't really get intense until about 8:00 P.M. I was in a lot of pain, so I got in the tub. Then I started getting sort of teary and saying I didn't know if I could handle this. I talked to the midwives and my husband and decided that I wanted to go to the hospital right away. On top of the pain, I had started being sick to my stomach, which really threw me off. They tell you about that in prenatal classes, but you think, That won't happen to me. I was sick at home and in the car on the way to the hospital. The student midwife was amazing: she stayed with us and kept her eyes on me the whole way to the hospital.

Being in the hospital couldn't have gone better. I really felt I was in a bubble of midwifery care in that setting. I didn't see any nurses, I didn't see any doctors. It was as though I had exchanged my bedroom for the hospital's bedroom. I didn't have to worry where I was standing or leaning or leaking on the floor. The bed seemed more comfortable than my own bed. I felt even more comfortable and secure than I had at home.

At the hospital, I became convinced that I could find the position that would make the pain go away. I couldn't, but I tried anyway. I was in the tub, I was out of the tub, I was leaning, I was on the bed. Then I went into transition. I wanted an epidural at that point, but all of a sudden I gave a huge push. This gave me an indication that it would be over soon. I was on my knees and leaning against the back of the bed. My second midwife got there for the pushing, and my son was born about half an hour later, at 12:20 A.M.

When I was in active labour, I had shut everything out. But all of a sudden my baby arrived, and I became aware of everybody else around me again. It felt blissful and overwhelming. The baby was so slippery that I was afraid he would roll off me. He was this amazing rosy, peachy pink colour. He looked radiant.

The grandparents came soon after he was born. I felt happy to be in the hospital then, because I had more control over my personal space. While I was having a couple of little stitches, they were out in the hallway. Then they came in and met the baby and took pictures while the midwives got me tea and toast. Then our families left, I had another bath, and my midwives helped me get dressed. Once we were ready, we left the hospital. We were home and tucked in by 4:00 A.M. The next morning, the midwives were back for a visit and a check-in.

—Nathalie, mother of one

If you have planned a hospital birth, the midwife or second attendant will most likely meet you at the hospital, instead of at your house. In some places, such as British Columbia, your second attendant will be an obstetric nurse on the floor at the time of your birth. The second attendant, whether a midwife, trained attendant or nurse, is necessary to ensure that there is one person devoted to you and one to the baby in the last stages of labour, at the birth and in the moments immediately following it. Having the encouragement of two midwives, or a midwife and her trained assistant, will also benefit you as you go through the final stages of exertion.

## Transition

Transition is the part of childbirth that takes you from the contraction stage to the stage when you push your baby out. The contractions in your uterus begin to change from opening the cervix to pushing downward through the cervix, and the effort involved is incredible. This stage is likely to be the most physically and emotionally demanding part of your labour. The good news is that at the end of it you will be fully dilated and your baby will be coming soon. Many women who felt that most of their labour was manageable say that in transition they felt they couldn't do it. If throwing up, crying uncontrollably, or yelling at your mate is going to happen, this will be the time for it.

Happily, transition is usually a relatively short part of your labour. Of course, you will probably have no idea how long this stage lasts and may not be able to identify it as transition, because you will be working so hard. Your midwives may be able to help you focus by reminding you that this is transition, that it will be over soon, and that this means your baby really is almost here. After transition passes, although labour is not over, many women say that at this point pushing seems like a huge relief.

## The Birth

### Pushing

The moment Miranda and her husband felt most grateful for their prenatal classes came during the first labour. Miranda was labouring alone in the bathroom when Jordan heard her make a low straining grunting noise. In the prenatal classes, the midwives had demonstrated the very distinct sound a woman makes when she pushes. Jordan was in another room, but that sound was so obviously the same one the midwives had demonstrated, he knew that if the midwives didn't come soon he would be catching his own baby. He called them to say they were needed immediately.

Some women become totally dilated and then have no real urge to push. This happens most often in cases where an epidural may have dulled the senses. But even women working without an epidural or other forms of pain relief sometimes say that they have to be told when to push. However, most times the body's signal that it is time to push is even more unmistakable. Your body pushes with incredible force, then the feeling subsides, and then it comes again. You may want to consciously push with the body's urges. Occasionally, the midwives may coach you about the most effective way to get through this. Sometimes some direction or a minor adjustment in your approach can make the pushing more effective.

In addition to an unstoppable urge to push, many women report a burning sensation as their outer body stretches to match the inner dilation. During most of the pushing phase, the sensation will diminish in between pushes. When it continues between pushes, the baby is probably very close to emerging.

*Position*

Just as finding the right positions can help you cope with labour and even help it progress, the positions you push in can help you move the baby out. Being in an upright position often speeds the baby's movement down and out, as gravity works with you. Some women assume a supported squat. In this position they are held on either side by midwives or support people. Others choose a birthing stool to get them into the same position. Reclining with your legs up close to your belly can be an effective way to open your pelvis and let yourself rest between pushes. Lying flat on your back can slow the baby's progress because you are fighting against gravity in this position. However, this stance is useful in situations where it is best to move the baby out more slowly. Some women also find that pushing on all fours is relatively comfortable and very effective.

Like everything else, the position that worked for someone else, or looked "right" in all the books, may not be the one that works for you in labour. In Sarah's first birth she used the birthing stool to get the baby to the crowning stage and then moved onto her side to slowly push the baby out. Miranda had thought she would push her baby out while remaining upright, but during labour she discovered that lying on her back or side was the position that felt comfortable, and it didn't interrupt the baby's progress. If a certain position is working for you and your baby, midwives will usually accommodate you by reaching and stretching in order to catch the baby, rather than getting you to move.

*Crowning*

With a first baby, before the baby emerges, there is usually a period where the head appears and then recedes. When the widest part of the baby's head remains at the opening of the vagina, this is called "crowning."

The midwives will tell you when they can see the baby's head and may ask you if you want to reach down and touch your son or daughter. Some women find this is just the encouragement they need to help the baby make the rest of the journey into the open.

The option of seeing the baby emerge is also wonderful and can have a similar effect. It can make you realize your effort is paying off and that your baby has almost arrived. You will find a mirror on your checklist of birth tools for just this purpose.

The pressure of the baby on your perineum (the skin and tissue of your pelvic floor) is intense in the moments right before birth. The midwives have techniques to minimize the impact on your perineum and to help you focus your energies. If you are giving birth out of the water, your midwives may apply hot compresses (or sometimes cold ones) and olive oil to your perineum to help the skin stretch without damage. Supporting the perineum in this way helps prevent your skin from tearing. The midwives will probably also help you to alter the power of your pushes so that your skin stretches to accommodate the baby's head instead of tearing to let it out. Easing up on these pushes while the baby crowns is sometimes referred to as "breathing the baby out."

Studies do not support the routine use of episiotomies. An episiotomy is a procedure in which the skin of the perineum is cut to give the baby a wider passage and to avoid tearing the mother's pelvic floor. Proponents of episiotomies will tell you that they discourage tears and heal better, but there is much evidence to the contrary. Imagine that your perineum is like fabric. While it is very difficult to rip a piece of cloth with only your two hands, the job becomes easy when you begin from an initial cut. When the perineum heals faster, it is more likely to stay healthy for the long term, which means fewer future problems like uterine prolapse and incontinence.

Midwives work to minimize tearing and only cut the perineum in emergency cases when the baby has to be brought those final centimetres out in a matter of seconds.

*Birth*

After the baby's head is out, there is usually a short pause as the baby rotates himself or herself to get the shoulders out, and then the baby slips out all the way. The midwives will either catch the baby or help the mother or her designated support person do this.

## Bonding and the First Moments

Many midwives do not routinely announce the sex of your baby, giving you or your support people the opportunity to do so. Many parents say that they were so busy marvelling at the baby that they didn't check the sex until a few minutes had passed. After the effort of the birth, this will probably seem like a relatively quiet, peaceful time. In most cases, the routine that follows the birth can unfold gradually, without a rush.

Midwives usually put your baby on your tummy and cover you both with blankets or towels, since the environment of the womb is almost always much warmer than the temperature in the birth room.

When the umbilical cord has stopped pulsating, the midwives will ask who would like to cut it, or will do so themselves if you wish. While you are snuggling with your baby, the midwives observe the baby's breathing and colour and watch for signs that you are ready to deliver the placenta. Though birthing the placenta may require a bit of pushing on your part, you may not even notice it coming while you look at your baby.

The midwives will assess your baby and assign an Apgar score at two intervals, at one minute and five minutes after the birth. The Apgar scale, named after physician Virginia Apgar, measures five factors (heart rate, respiration, muscle tone, reflex and colour) and assigns them a total score out of 10. Later, the midwives will also weigh your baby, take his or her temperature, and do a full newborn exam. Most of these checks will take place right beside you. However, if you are in a hospital setting, you or your designated support person can stay with the baby while he or she is weighed and checked in or out of the birthing room.

The midwives will also make sure that you are not losing too much blood and will check the condition of your perineum. If they find any tearing there, they will repair it with stitching if necessary.

The midwives will also examine the placenta to make sure it is intact. If fragments of the placenta are left attached to the uterus they can cause infection. They will offer you the opportunity to take a look at the placenta too—but rest assured that it is not a requirement! Though it may not sound immediately appealing, seeing the organ that fed your baby for nine months is a pretty amazing thing. If you give birth in hospital or in a birth centre, the midwives will ask you whether you want the staff to dispose of the placenta or whether you wish to take it home. If you are at home, you can keep it or throw it away. In some areas it may be illegal to throw it in the garbage, so check with your midwife first. Most people who keep the placenta will freeze it in a grocery bag. Later they will bury it and sometimes plant something for the baby on top of it, such as a rose bush or a tree.

### The First Feeding

The midwives will help clean you up and will get you into clean sheets. When everyone is comfortable, they will help you put your baby to the breast for the first time. Your baby may or may not be enthusiastic about nursing, and you will probably need to make a few attempts before you get him or her to latch on. Do not be alarmed about this. Whether it is easy or hard to feed your baby the first time, nursing is a skill that needs to be learned by mother and baby. It does not need to be perfect the first time. As you get to know each other, you will both become more proficient at it. (More information on breastfeeding appears in Chapter 11.)

In the first little while after birth, nursing begins the process of helping your uterus contract and stimulates milk production. Babies don't usually need fluid in the first few hours after birth, but the liquid that your body is already producing is very important. It's called colostrum, and it contains all sorts of disease-fighting properties that will benefit your child. If your little one doesn't take too much in for the first couple of hours, don't panic. The midwives will help you to monitor how much your child is getting and make sure that he or she is well hydrated. Your body will start producing milk in about three to five days.

## Going Home, Getting Rest

For those mothers who have had their babies in hospital or at a birth centre, the trip home usually happens within a few hours of birth. If you have had complications during labour or birth, or if you do not feel up to the move at this time, you can arrange to stay longer at the hospital. Most mothers, though, find that immediately following the birth, they experience a boost of energy that allows them to make the trip home before they need that first, long post-labour sleep. If you are already at home, the biggest trip you will probably need to make is to the bathroom.

Many women and their partners or other personal support people describe the period after birth as a "high." Realizing what you have accomplished can be a wonderful feeling. If you are up to making phone calls and taking pictures, it's a great time to do it. But it can also be a time of simple quiet wonder. Don't worry if your baby cries a lot immediately after birth, since some babies are very vocal, and the quiet time will follow.

One way or another, it is very important to try to get rest within a few hours of the birth. Eventually the high will subside, and you will need rest after your supreme effort. Your baby will also be exhausted from his or her hard work. Best to capitalize on that exhaustion and sleep while you can! Though many babies remain relatively sleepy for a while after birth, others will be wide awake soon after. Since you can't predict your baby's temperament yet, it's best to rest while you have the opportunity.

## Changes and Challenges

Every birth has its challenges, but sometimes the actual birth radically differs from the one you had planned. Your midwives will help you to adapt to any new conditions by providing you with information and support.

### Staying at Home

Precipitous births are more frequent in sitcoms than in real life, but situations in which babies arrive much more quickly than expected do happen sometimes. Occasionally a planned hospital birth will turn into an unplanned homebirth. Parents planning a birth with midwives are probably better able to deal with this turn of events than those who had planned to labour and give birth in hospital with the help of a medical team. Since midwifery clients usually plan to do their labouring at home, there are often some supplies on hand, and the midwives are the only professionals specifically trained to help women birth at home. Of course, a major shift in thinking is required if your planned hospital birth ends up happening in your own bed, but in a quick birthing situation you will probably be too focused on labour to think so much about location.

If your labour is progressing so quickly that it seems the baby will arrive soon, call your midwives so that they can talk you through what is happening, and tell you how soon they will be there and whether you should call an ambulance.

**A surprise homebirth**

The birth was the best part by far. We were planning a hospital birth. This was part of the comfort-zone plan. I thought homebirths had some element of hippiedom in them that I was not searching for. Besides, I know where the dust bunnies live. Well, you know what they say about best-laid plans.

When Carolyn told me she thought her water had broken, I was pretty calm. I was calm when I called our midwife. When Carolyn's first contraction hit, I was calm. When the second one hit about a minute later, I felt confused. It wasn't until I called the midwife again and she said she was coming right over that the idea our baby might be born at home entered my mind. The irony is that I do not remember discussing precipitous births with either of our midwives. The plan seemed to be going out the window. It was completely shot when our midwife said the facility we had planned to use, a smaller community hospital, was under quarantine due to an outbreak of chicken pox. Afterwards, Carolyn said there was no way we would have gotten her in a car, even if the hospital was open. She was right. We would never have made it. Esther was going to be born at home.

Our primary midwife got to our home about 40 minutes before the birth. Legally, she required another midwife to be present and our backup midwife arrived with about 10 minutes to spare. I might be seeing the past through rose-coloured glasses, but I think we all felt pretty calm at that point. They had their gear set up very quickly. I offered to boil water (because all these years you've seen on TV some poor dad being sent off to boil water and fetch warm blankets) but was glad when they said all we needed was some towels. I had stopped worrying about the dust bunnies now. I was with experienced people performing a safe, healthy birth. It felt great.

—*Chris, father of two*


*Transferring to Hospital*

If you have had your heart set on a homebirth or having your baby at a birth centre, making the choice to move to hospital during labour may involve a difficult sacrifice. Though the majority of planned homebirths or birth centre births with midwives are accomplished without a move to hospital (even in the case of first-time mothers), there are times when the mother and her midwives will decide that hospital technology offers the mom a better chance of birthing her baby without a C-section. Most transfers to hospital do not result from emergencies but are an attempt to assist the mother as she goes through a particularly long or difficult labour. After many hours of work that's yielded little progress, an epidural and labour augmentation with oxytocin may give the mother an opportunity to continue with renewed energy.

Many women admit they fear that they will lose the respect of their support people and midwives if they change their plans in labour and decide to give birth in hospital instead of at home. Changes in plans should never be considered a failure. While the midwives want to help you give birth in as natural a way as possible, they have attended many, many births in a wide range of different circumstances. Combine this with their thorough knowledge of your health and your hopes for your labour and birth. They will not only be able to help you determine what physical and emotional resources you need, but also will be able to help you assess your situation and make measured projections about your progress. If you decide together that you need the kind of help that is only available at the hospital, then you should be assured of their continued support and respect. Midwives across the country have told us that their primary aim is to provide respectful care no matter what kind of birth they attend and to help women birth with confidence. That confidence stems from doing a difficult job well. There is no "right" way to give birth; nor is there a "right" way to cope with labour and the other challenges associated with birth. Every birth is different; some present greater challenges than others. The midwives' goal is to help you to accomplish the best birth for you and your baby in your particular circumstances.

**Midwives support Jane's change of plans**

I was too exhausted and tired to go on. My partner and I talked with our midwives about the possibility of going to the hospital. When I told my midwife that I did want to go, she was so supportive. I think now of the two days and nights of sleep she lost as she helped me labour at home, and she never once grumbled or appeared frustrated. All I ever felt from them was support and encouragement.

—Jane, mother of two

*Interventions*

Of course, there are times when the decision to move locations or seek interventions becomes a necessity rather than a choice, in order to ensure the safety of mother and baby. Be assured that these occasions occur relatively infrequently. Should they occur, your midwives will assist you to get the care you need.

### Finding beauty in a different birth experience

I found a new sense of peace when I realized that my baby's head was closest to my heart. Suddenly I appreciated her breech position rather than resenting it. Despite this "abnormal" position, she continued to grow, move and hiccup within the nourishing environment of my uterus, completely oblivious to the risks of her upcoming birth.

Then I realized that this birth was not just about me. I had been completely focused on the birthing experience as a rite of passage, a time when a woman learns of her true power. But apparently the birth gods feel there is a deeper, very different lesson for me to learn from this birth. I think they are concerned about my seemingly false illusion of motherhood (and perhaps of life). I was fortunate to have an easy conception and an incredibly smooth and healthy pregnancy. Until now, I believed that as long as I did all the "right" things everything would be perfect. Now I had to change my idea of perfection.

The Caesarean was beautiful. The birth gods smiled on us that day. They sent their angels into that operating room. Everyone was so kind and gentle. When it was time for Ayla to be born, the nurses dropped the sheet and we saw her beautiful body emerge from my womb. She was placed in my arms within moments of her birth, and in my arms she stayed.

I lost out on the birthing experience, but I gained a beautiful daughter, whom I respect deeply. Ayla taught me that birth, much like life, cannot be "planned" or "controlled." She taught me that in the pursuit of our dreams, we must know when it is time to surrender. I feel as though I understand Ayla better because of our experience together. I look forward to watching her grow into a beautiful woman who will one day have her own birthing experiences. I hope I can be there to help her to listen to her body . . . and her baby.

—*Patti, mother of one*

No one plans to have a baby that decides to manoeuvre into a difficult position in the birth canal, or to labour without dilating, for example, but these situations do occur. What will happen in the event you or your baby needs the type of assistance that lies beyond the midwives' scope of practice?

If you are at home or in a birth centre, the midwives will help you move to the hospital. They will either get you there in a car or call an ambulance. The midwives will then accompany you to the hospital. When you arrive, they will get you the care you need by consulting with the appropriate medical personnel—namely, anesthetists, obstetricians or pediatricians. If a genuine emergency is underway, the medical staff will prepare whatever interventions are necessary as soon as they are informed of the situation by the midwives, who will call from the birth centre or your home.

### Marielle's midwife keeps her informed

We were at the birth centre and everything had been going fine. I was very solitary, but I felt supported by my partner and my midwife's presence. She was very hands-off, just letting me go through it. Then at the end, when we had meconium staining in the amniotic fluid (when the baby has a bowel movement in utero), my midwife was very honest. She looked me straight in the eye and said, "This is serious. This is what you have . . . These are the potential problems . . ." She was direct and clear, she was exposing the situation, giving it reality. She made us feel in control when facing potential problems.

—*Marielle, mother of one*

In most situations, midwives will remain as advocates and intermediaries for their clients, even when care is transferred to medical personnel. In some areas, medical interventions, such as an epidural, an induction or an intravenous drip, fall within the midwives' scope of practice, so your midwives may be able to remain your primary caregivers. Determining the midwives' continuing role occurs in consultation with medical staff, who will remain on hand for backup assistance should the need arise. In other cases, midwives may be able to transfer care to a physician temporarily while the doctor provides the medical assistance, and then the doctor will hand care of the mother and baby back to the midwives. If the interventions required do not fall within the midwives' scope of practice, the midwives will almost always remain with you as labour support persons.

How such arrangements will play out between midwives and medical staff depends partly on the status of midwives in your province and partly on the working relationships between the midwives and the medical staff on duty. In a best-case scenario, the transfer of care in a hospital setting should be seamless, and the midwives should be there to offer you continued support and guidance so you know that you and your baby are receiving the best possible care.

### Midwife support after transfer of care

Through my tears and frustration at the hospital, my midwife stuck by my side as they prepped me for a C-section. I remember her words of wisdom were that birth was humbling and made you face your fears. Unfortunately, my greatest fears had been doctors and hospitals. At that moment, I felt so glad I had a midwife because she was the only one allowed in into the operating room with me. Not even my partner could come in until after they had operated. My sense of failure was deep but fleeting as I was greeted with the healthy cry of my 10-pound baby boy.

—*Kelly, mother of one*

Most midwifery clients do not approach their birth expecting a C-section. However, most midwives have considerable experience with such situations and will therefore be able to support you during this operation. Midwives are often allowed to accompany their clients into the operating room and will observe the process so that they can tell you what happened afterward. They may also be able to help care for your baby while you are stitched up, and will keep your support people informed of what is happening.

*Support in Hospital*

If there are factors that keep you in the hospital for a few days after the birth (perhaps you have had a C-section or your baby requires additional care), you can expect your midwives to support you during your hospital stay by being just a phone call away.

**Calling the hospital for advice**

On the day that our baby was born we really wanted to go home after several hours. We had both rested and our midwives had gone home. The hospital staff were concerned about some blood tests that remained to be done. So we called our midwife to seek her advice. Having her there to talk to made all the difference. We felt confident that we could get the care we needed and still be in our home with our baby.

—*Mike, father of one*

If you have had a C-section, you will need to stay in the hospital for several days. You will need help because the incision may make it difficult to sit or hold your baby. While you remain in hospital, your midwife will probably visit you and will keep in touch by phone. She may be able to explain hospital practices, discuss the birth and prepare you for the time when you and your baby go home.

If your baby needs special care, your midwife will take an active role in helping you find the appropriate specialists. Your midwife will also offer you the support you need to ensure that breastfeeding remains an option, even if your baby can't nurse right away.

Many families whose babies did not arrive in a straightforward manner credit their midwives with making the birth and bonding process as normal as possible.

### ◎ *If You Want to Read More . . .*

*The Birth Book*, by William Sears and Martha Sears (Boston: Little, Brown and Company, 1994).

*The Complete Book of Pregnancy and Childbirth* (new ed.), by Sheila Kitzinger (London: Dorling Kindersley Limited, 1996).

*A Husband-Coached Childbirth*, by Robert A. Bradley (Sherman Oaks, California: Bantam, 1996).

*One Mother to Another*, by Winifred Wallace Hunsburger (Saskatoon, Saskatchewan: Fifth House Publishers, 1992).

*Wise Woman Herbal for the Childbearing Year*, by Susun S. Weed (Woodstock, New York: Ash Tree Publishing, 1986).

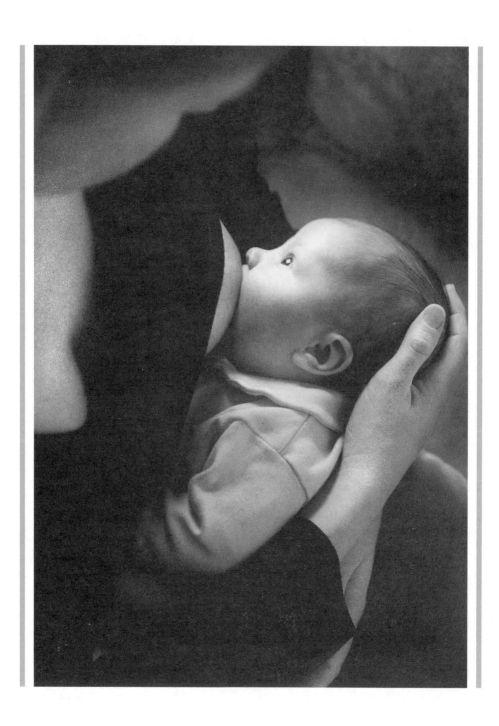

## Eleven

### Early Days

**Appreciating midwifery postpartum**

When I found out I was pregnant, I knew I would opt for a midwife for a number of reasons, both political and personal. None of them had to do with what would happen after the birth—during pregnancy, who can imagine life after birth? In hindsight, the reason I was so happy with my midwife had much more to do with her work after the birth of my baby than before.

—*Kelly, mother of one*

Many parents say that the time they most appreciated their midwifery care was during the first few days at home with a newborn. It's an old truism that babies come with no instruction manual. Though you can surround yourself with reading material about how to deal with *a* baby, none of it will tell you about how to deal with your own. The first few days of being a new parent are ones of intense discovery. Having the midwives nearby to answer practical questions can help you focus on learning about your new son or daughter.

Just as the midwives supported you in your many decisions as an expectant mother, they will support you after the birth. Midwives are not there to tell you how to parent but to help you get the help you need to parent your own way—even if you are not sure what that way is yet.

### A lifeline of support

I can't say enough about the support I received from the midwives afterwards. I had more support from them than I did from my family. Just the feeling that I could call if I needed to, helped me. There was no way I would have had that lifeline if I hadn't chosen midwives. With my first baby, I needed them so much in the pregnancy. With my second, I most appreciated them afterwards.

*—Jessica, mother of two*

For most people, the first days of a baby's life do not resemble the sort of pastel portrait of mother and child one might find on a Hallmark greeting card. The maternal bliss thing does happen but usually not right away. A baby's needs are pretty basic: food, sleep, comfort. Simple needs but also absolute ones. Meeting them is more than a full-time job, and you will have to tap into your physical and mental strength. Anticipating that the work of feeding, changing and comforting your infant will be all-absorbing will make things easier for both you and your baby.

### Countless questions

When I came home from the hospital five days after giving birth, my legs were still twice their normal size. But once I got home, we were pretty preoccupied with looking after our daughter. And the midwives' follow-up was amazing. They'd walk through the door and I'd have half an hour's worth of questions for them. I don't know how other couples live without that kind of support.

*—Barb, mother of one*

It is quite common for new mothers to wonder, What have I done all day? Unfortunately, it is also quite common for mothers of infants to be asked by well-meaning people, "What have you done all day?" Miranda suggest that people in her postpartum group reply: "I nurtured a life. You?"

## Your Baby

*Feeding*

With the help of public service announcements and a shift in cultural norms, Canadian society is realizing that "Breast Is Best." Breastfeeding provides your baby with more nutrition than any formula, no matter how carefully concocted. Recent studies have shown that breast milk has long-lasting health effects in many areas. For example, it reduces the incidence of allergies, ear infections, lower respiratory infections and urinary tract infections in children. There is also a decreased incidence of bacterial meningitis. Breastfeeding develops the facial muscles in ways that sucking a bottle nipple cannot. A child uses these muscles when learning how to talk. Breastfeeding helps the mother's body, too, by increasing uterine contractions, which help organs settle back into place more quickly, allowing for a speedier recovery. Over several months, breastfeeding also helps many women lose the weight they acquired while pregnant.

Many people see breastfeeding as "natural." Expectant mothers and onlookers alike often equate *natural* with *easy*, as in "it comes naturally." The reality of breastfeeding is that it is a skill that needs to be learned by mother and baby alike. Yes, there are new mothers and babies for whom breastfeeding is an easy experience, but many, many mothers and babies find it a challenge. Within a few weeks or months, can you tell the difference between mothers and infants who started off easily and those who didn't? No. In some cases you will find your most committed nursers among those moms and kids who didn't have an easy start.

In the hour or two that follow your baby's birth, the midwives will assist you in putting your baby to the breast. For most people, the trick here is getting the baby to "latch on" properly. The proper latch is essential to good nursing because it allows the baby to get enough food and preserves the mother's nipples. For a proper latch, the baby needs a wide mouth and a tongue that is flat in the mouth. He or she has to take the nipple and the areola surrounding the nipple into the mouth to be able to suck effectively.

Usually, moms and babies go through a period of trial and error, so do not be alarmed if things don't click right away. Similarly, the baby who seems to take to the breast naturally on the first feeding, may surprise you at 3:00 A.M. by having no idea how to make it work. Many attempts over many days may be required to really get the hang of it.

A baby needs to nurse frequently—some moms would say, almost constantly—during the first few days of life. Crying newborns should be offered the breast as a first solution, and newborns should go no more than two to three hours without feeding. However, one long sleep a day (five to six hours) is safe, provided your baby is already well hydrated. At this stage, your baby is learning feeding habits, getting essential nutrients and much-needed liquid. A lot of sleepy babies need to be woken to feed, and then there are those who seem to nurse without even taking a break to sleep. Your baby will reveal his or her own unique personality pretty quickly.

Though your midwives pack up their equipment and leave within a few hours of your baby's birth, they will come back several times over the next few days and will be available by phone on a 24-hour basis. If you think that your baby is not getting enough milk, or if you are worried because you and your baby cannot get a good latch, the midwives will be able to coach you. If the problem persists, your midwives may refer you to a lactation consultant or a breastfeeding clinic.

The midwives will be able to show you the signs that the baby is sucking properly and help you get the best position for holding the baby. They will teach you other ways to determine whether the baby is getting enough milk and will help you monitor your particular baby's intake. As the midwives will tell you, one of the best ways to judge what your baby is taking in is by assessing what he or she is putting out. By day six your newborn should have at least six wet diapers a day. See the end of this chapter for resources on breastfeeding.

*Cord care*

Before your baby's cord is cut, the midwives will clamp it with a metal or a plastic clamp or a cloth tie. When the cord dries out in a day or two, the midwives will remove the clamp, leaving a little dried-up stump of skin. This may fall off within a few days or a couple of weeks. Some parents find the stump a little worrisome or gross. If you're careful not to let clothing rub it or not to get it very wet, it shouldn't bother you or the baby. Sometimes a wet cord can get a bit smelly, but the midwives will show you how to clean it, if this becomes an issue. Most often, it is best to leave the stump alone. Many parents almost forget it is there until, one diaper change, they suddenly see the baby's belly button.

*Diapering*

In the first few days of his life, your baby should have about two or three wet diapers per day. In these early days your baby will have very black sticky stools. This is called meconium and is the product of digested amniotic fluid. This will change to a liquidy orange or yellow colour as your baby begins to digest milk. After the first few days, your baby will have from six to eight wet diapers a day. He or she will also probably have two to five bowel movements each day. All of these signs indicate that your baby is getting enough to eat. Frequent changes of diapers in the first week will help you to learn about your baby. Some parents find it helpful to keep a log book of baby changes (and feedings too) so they can give an accurate account of the baby's progress and health to the midwives.

**Assessing a wet diaper**

An easy way to feel the weight of a wet disposable diaper is to pour 2–4 tablespoons of water in a dry diaper.

—*La Leche League International*

*Dressing*

In the last trimester of pregnancy, the baby's movements *in utero* are very restricted, and many babies feel quite frightened when their limbs are suddenly free. The midwives can show you how to swaddle your baby in a blanket to feel safe and secure. Sarah's midwife is an expert swaddler and would always leave the baby looking like a nicely wrapped present. Sarah's partner became quite adept too, rolling and tucking the baby in to his great satisfaction. He would still be swaddling them today if they would let him! Try as she might, Sarah could never quite get the hang of it, which didn't matter, as her baby was happy with all attempts.

Some babies spend weeks tightly bundled. Babies who like this feeling will feel quite shocked when they are naked, and may object strongly to being completely undressed. You can help by undressing them in stages: changing a diaper while they are wearing a T-shirt, for example.

Not long ago, conventional wisdom dictated that babies needed to be dressed warmly, no matter the season. Now we know that overheating is a bigger concern. A baby who feels cold will usually cry, which will alert you to the problem. The fussing actually helps him warm himself as he moves around and cries. A baby who is overheated is actually at greater risk of SIDS (sudden infant death syndrome). An easy way to tell if your baby is too hot is to feel her hands. Babies' hands tend to be cool, because their bodies are just learning to circulate blood efficiently. If your baby's hands feel really warm, then you should consider taking off some layers of clothing till you've cooled her down. A good way to judge your baby's clothing needs is to dress her as you would yourself, then add one layer.

*Sleeping*

Some babies sleep most of the time. Some babies hardly ever sleep. There is very little, if anything, you can do about your infant's sleep patterns. The best bet is to heed the old saying that the mother should "sleep when the baby sleeps." Of course, this is easier to accomplish when you have only one child.

A sleepy baby will sleep just about anywhere. Some parents like to have the baby in his or her own room, others want the baby next to them in bed. Whatever suits you is just fine, provided the baby is in a safe space and you can nurse easily. Wherever they are sleeping, babies should be on a firm mattress (unless you are the mattress!), with no opportunity for their faces to be covered by bedding. Again, remember that they should not be too warm. Repeated studies have shown that putting babies on their backs to sleep substantially reduces the chance of SIDS.

### Bathing

Some parents opt to bathe their babies soon after they are born; others like to leave the birth residue on the baby's skin for a while. Whichever your choice, your baby will need to be cleaned eventually. "How dirty can they be?" is one of those infamous new parent questions that gets answered pretty quickly with one spectacular poo or when you realize that that cute little crease is hiding dead skin (that smells and makes the surrounding area red and sore).

Babies don't need soaps and lotions: a little water or olive oil will help clear away dead skin and dirty diaper residue without irritating their skin. You can wipe your baby down with a washcloth. You also might put him or her in some sort of small tub, or take him or her into a pleasantly warm bath with you. Some babies love the feel of water, while others don't even want to be undressed. At Miranda's house, the baby's first bath with Dad was a ritual that one child loved and the other hated—so for the one, it ended pretty quickly. If your baby likes the feel of the tub, it can be a great quiet time for both parent and infant. Some mothers report that their babies who have difficulty latching sometimes breastfeed without a fuss while having a warm bath with mom.

*Crying*

Babies start smiling intentionally at about four to six weeks—or "just in time" as the old joke goes, meaning that after weeks of caring for such a demanding creature, parents need to feel they are appreciated. Real cooing and babbling doesn't start for several months. In the first few days and weeks of life, crying is your baby's sole means of communicating needs. At first, all your baby's crying will sound the same to you, but soon you'll become an expert at interpreting the code.

Some babies are more naturally quiet, while some are expressive. How much your baby cries does not reflect on your skills as a parent. What you want to do is to respond as best you can to your baby's needs.

If your baby feels uncomfortable in any way, he or she will probably cry. That discomfort can be caused by hunger, being too hot or too cold, being held in an uncomfortable position, or being afraid or tired. The tears may also mean your baby has gas or his or her clothes are too tight. As you get better acquainted with your new child, you will probably develop a checklist that you run through unconsciously: *Are you hungry? Are you wet? Is the sun in your eyes? Do you want to be held? Do you want to be put down?* Remember that your baby is the best judge of needs. You may have fed him or her for 40 minutes just an hour ago, but if a baby's hungry, it's hungry.

A baby who can't be comforted by practical means such as breastfeeding may settle down if you sing or rock the baby. You could also go for a walk or drive with the infant. Some babies get so worked up about not latching on to the breast right away that they scream themselves into a fit that makes latching impossible. In this case, it is probably better to try to find an alternative means of comfort so that the baby can calm down and then try again.

Most often, you will know you've identified the source of the discomfort when the baby settles down. Your reward is a silent, peaceful baby. Other times, your baby will cry no matter what you do. This distresses most parents. You want your baby to be content, and you are doing your best to help the infant feel comfortable. Consult with your midwives to see if they can bring an outside perspective to the situation or suggest another approach. But if you have run through your checklist and all your tricks, sometimes all you can do is hold your little one until the crying stops.

If you can, enlist help to rock the baby so that you can refuel your enthusiasm with a break. A calm parent is more likely to be responsive and patient, to ride out this particular storm. At this point, it is good to think about ways to comfort yourself so that you can continue to provide your baby with the love that he or she needs.

## Circumcision

If you choose to circumcise your son for reasons based on faith, you will probably have the procedure done as part of a ceremony in the couple of weeks following his birth. If you are considering circumcision for reasons other than religion, you will have some decisions to make. First of all, it is important to know that most infant boys are not circumcised these days. So if you are concerned about future locker room taunts, he will be in good company whether or not you choose the procedure. Most medical bodies no longer recommend routine circumcision, and your son can easily be taught how to take care of his foreskin so that cleanliness is not an issue.

In most provinces, doctors perform circumcision for a fee, as it is no longer considered a medically necessary service. Circumcisions are not done immediately after birth; you may need to bring your baby to the hospital or to a doctor's office for the procedure. Your midwives may be able to recommend a *mohel* (rhymes with foil) who would also do the procedure for a fee. Mohels are specialists in circumcision because they perform them on Jewish boys at their bris ceremony.

## Tests and Treatments for Baby

In the hours and days that follow your baby's birth, your midwives will perform a number of procedures that are generally considered routine or required by public health regulations. Your midwife will inform you of the latest research on each test and the local requirements for administration in the last few appointments before birth. She will point you in the direction of further information, if you want it.

## Vitamin K

One of these procedures is the administration of vitamin K, usually by injection. Vitamin K helps newborns' blood clot. Babies are born with less vitamin K than adults, and in most instances this would not pose a problem. However, one rare condition called hemorrhagic disease of the newborn is eradicated by the routine use of vitamin K injections for all babies. For vitamin K to be effective, it needs to be administered in the first hours after birth.

## Eye prophylaxis

Antibiotic eye drops are also administered to newborns within two hours of birth, as required by law. The antibiotics may help prevent infection in the newborn's eyes, which could be a result of bacteria picked up in the passage through the birth canal. The kinds of bacteria that can create problems are those caused by infections such as gonorrhea and chlamydia. These bacteria, which can be asymptomatic in women, can cause blindness in newborn babies.

## Phenylketonuria (PKU) and Thyroid Test

Phenylketonuria (PKU) is a genetic problem that interferes with the metabolism of the important essential amino acid phenylalanine. If this amino acid cannot be metabolized, it will become toxic to brain tissue and cause brain damage. When diagnosed early, this condition is treatable. The PKU test is a blood test, usually done within days of birth. For the PKU test, your midwife will prick the baby's heel to draw a small amount of blood, which is then applied to a special paper and sent to a lab.

This same test also screens for hypothyroidism, which can cause both mental and physical developmental abnormalities. Early diagnosis and treatment prevents these problems.

## Mom

Just because you are working hard to take care of your new baby doesn't mean that you shouldn't take care of yourself too. Parents are a baby's best chance for everything. It's a huge responsibility, and the healthier you are the better able you will be to take on the challenge.

### Mothering the mother

My favourite parts of midwife-attended births come after the birth. At this time, the midwives provide mothering to me and reassurance, which I don't get from family members. They allow us to be with our newborn, performing the necessary tasks as unobtrusively as possible. During labour, it has always been my husband and me, with them as bystanders, monitoring what we can't know. I don't draw on their strength at that time, but our own. It is an intimate time for us. And they let us be private. After the birth, I welcome their wisdom. I am less focused on the task and more self-conscious and nervous. How much bleeding is too much? What if he won't nurse? Should the cord look like that? I feel shaky: is my blood pressure O.K.? I've been through the wringer, but they settle me in bed and marvel at my babe and praise me and my husband for the great work we have done. I need to be mothered and the midwives do it so well.

*—Susan, mother of three*

### *Recovering*

The story about how women used to squat in a field, give birth and keeping working is a myth. Most societies have highly developed rituals for caring for a mother who has recently given birth. In many places in the world, women are given special herb baths, massages, and special strengthening and purifying drinks. Women are often not expected to immediately rejoin larger society but rather remain secluded for anywhere from 3 to 40 days. Typically, in North American society, almost all the attention falls on the infant, while the mother's equally great needs are largely ignored.

Choosing midwifery is an excellent way to combat that effect, whether or not mothers know it when they opt for this type of care. Midwives will monitor your progress in the days and weeks after birth, noting how your body and emotions are recovering from the birth itself and how you are responding to the demands of mothering. One of the greatest services that midwives provide is the time and inclination to listen.

Most midwives will frequently remind you that you need rest to recover, but we'd like to reiterate this. Your body has gone through huge changes in nine months, culminating in a great athletic effort to birth your baby. If you had a C-section, your body has done its nine months and undergone major surgery. Whatever your history, your body needs the time to stage a comeback. However, it's now under new management with incredibly long hours and demands.

Rest whenever you can, no matter how bizarre the timing seems to you. If the baby is sleeping, or your partner is walking the baby around the block, take advantage of the time. You may think you will feel better if you use the time to put away the diapers, but you will not. Someone else can tidy and cook or order pizza. Only you can rest for yourself.

Some women feel overcome with energy in the first few days after they give birth, but trying to get out too soon or take on too much is not usually a good idea. Gardening two days after your baby is born might feel great at the time, but there may be serious repercussions. Your body needs rest to produce milk in sufficient supply to feed your baby, and its ability to fight off infection is a great deal stronger if you've done your time in bed or reclining on the couch. Also, in the days right after birth, gravity is not your friend! Your uterus shrinks from the size of a watermelon to that of a grapefruit. As this happens, all your other organs move back into their original places—or try to. Many conditions that plague older women—such as a prolapsed uterus or bladder, which makes them incontinent—might be traced back to their insufficient recovery time after their children were born. Urinary continence is a good thing. Stay in bed.

### Bleeding

Now you know what those industrial-sized pads on the drugstore shelf are for. For the first few days after your baby is born, you will bleed quite heavily. Over the first week, the bleeding will gradually taper off, and somewhere between a week and six weeks, it will stop. The length of time that a woman bleeds and how much she bleeds depends on the individual. What you need to keep track of is the consistency of the bleeding. If you have been changing your pad every couple of hours, then suddenly have to get three new pads in an hour, call your midwife immediately.

In the first little while after birth, you may pass some blood clots. Seeing a large clot can be quite disturbing if you aren't expecting it. But clotting, which is just pooled and congealed blood, is quite normal. If you pass several clots, monitor yourself closely and report to your midwife.

### Healing

Many women experience tearing of the perineum, or pelvic floor, while pushing their babies out, and the tears often require some stitching. Your pelvic area may also be swollen from your effort. Putting ice packs on the tender area (you can use packages of frozen peas or corn) will go a long way to lessen your discomfort and speed the healing. Other treatments include sitz baths—baths of warm water, which sometimes include herbs. Your midwife will check to make sure that everything is healing well and that no infections have set in.

Sometimes, the touch of urine on your perineum can also be uncomfortable at first. Filling a squirt bottle with warm water and pouring it over your perineum while you pee can help dilute the urine and ease the burning sensation.

Many women will get hemorrhoids for the first time when they are pregnant. This can come as quite a shock. Learning how to treat this condition early on, rather than ignoring it in the hopes it will just go away, will save you a lot of discomfort in the long run. There will often be a flare-up right after birth because of all the straining involved in pushing your baby out. Sitz baths will help, as will commercial preparations designed to soothe and shrink hemorrhoids. Eating lots of fruits and vegetables and drinking lots of water or taking a stool softener will help as everything inside settles back into place.

*Milk*

In the first few days after birth, your breastfeeding baby will not be getting straight milk, but a substance called colostrum. It's sometimes referred to as liquid gold because of its makeup and yellowy colour. Colostrum is very important because it contains carbohydrates, protein and antibodies. It can be easily digested by your newborn and a little of this highly concentrated substance goes a long way. Colostrum also functions as a laxative, making it easier for your baby to pass those first sticky stools.

Somewhere between days three and five, your milk will come in. In some cases it trickles in slowly, resulting in a tawny mixture of colostrum and milk. In other cases it seems to come in overnight. This can cause your breasts to jump a cup size or two in a matter of hours, which can be alarming. Your breasts may become very hot and hard. It is extremely important during this time to nurse frequently or express milk by hand or with a pump to avoid breast engorgement. Sometimes your breasts can be so full at this stage that your baby may find it difficult to get a good latch. The milk can also come rushing out, as if from a fountain, which may overwhelm your baby. This stage doesn't usually last for very long. Over time, your baby will regulate the amount of milk in your body by signalling his or her needs. As the baby sucks, milk production is stimulated, creating just the right supply for the demand.

Most women produce an adequate amount of milk, but your body needs rest, a steady supply of replacement liquid and good nutrition to do so. If you and your midwives determine that your milk supply is insufficient, take to your bed, drink a large glass of water every time you put the baby to your breast, and have other people bring you healthy meals and snacks frequently. There are also natural supplements and prescription drugs for the infrequent times when supply cannot be adjusted to demand. Refer to one of the recommended readings at the end of this chapter for more expert and comprehensive advice on breastfeeding.

**Working through breastfeeding challenges**

I think that I may have given up on breastfeeding if it hadn't been for the midwives. You read about it. Then you are confronted with this child and this breast and you know that they are supposed to fit together, but you don't know how. It just seems like this strange, otherworldly thing to be doing. My baby wasn't opening his mouth, and I didn't know what to do. My midwife just came in and said, "Here's the plan. Do you want to persevere?" and we replied, yes. Then she said, "The baby needs to learn how to eat. That's his job. And here's how we're going to work on it."

The next few days were a blur of pumping and feeding and trying to nurse. But I was still able to be very happy, because I knew that our midwives were taking care of everything, and I trusted them. I knew that if they said the baby was doing O.K., then he was, and it would all work out. Eventually it did.

—*Nathalie, mother of one*

*Nursing Troubles*

As we mentioned earlier, nursing represents a challenge for some mothers and some babies. That challenge can come in the form of concerns about milk supply; sore breasts; babies who nurse almost constantly, allowing little time for the mom to sleep; or babies who seem to have trouble latching on.

If your baby can't quite get the hang of nursing, your midwives will help you to keep trying until the baby catches on. If the learning process is going to be a long one—more than a day or two—the midwives will be able to help you determine whether interim measures are needed: like pumping milk from your breasts and feeding the baby with a little tube. Because the sucking reflex is one of the last skills babies master *in utero*, those born a few weeks early often take longer to accomplish latching on.

**Breastfeeding perseverance and success**

After various nurses, lactation consultants and midwives manipulated my breast and Aidan's mouth to help them fit together, everyone agreed I would need to pump to get the milk into him. I began to pump every drop of colostrum and milk I could. Aidan was finger-fed with a tube so that he wouldn't get used to a bottle—in the hope that he would one day nurse. We got plenty of advice and pressure about supplementing, but we stuck with our midwife, who said he was fine with whatever I pumped. On our first night at home, our midwife spent a lot of time with us trying to teach Aidan to nurse. She came over every day to weigh him and try again.

I remember the day Aidan finally latched. He was eight days old and we were sitting around the living room chatting quietly. I thought I would try just for a second and if it didn't work, he could be tube-fed. There would be no tears, no fights, no emotional strain tonight. Amazingly, he latched on and nursed for 20 minutes! I sat quietly, trying not to draw attention to him lest he stop. He is now a year old and hasn't stopped yet!

What I loved about having a midwife was the support I received after my baby was born. Because of my C-section I didn't have the dream homebirth I had hoped for, and my midwife didn't catch my son as he was born. But she helped to catch him in another way, by encouraging us to continue waiting until he was ready to nurse. This was the most difficult part of birthing Aidan. His resistance was so strong; he screamed so loud when offered the breast that putting a bottle in his mouth would have been so easy. It took enormous strength and support to keep pumping, trying and tube-feeding, knowing that breast milk would truly be best for him in the end. No one but a midwife would have seen me through that.

—*Kelly, mother of one*

With any nursing challenge, expert advice, stop-gap measures, patience and a sense of humour seem to be the recipe for ultimate success. In

Miranda's postpartum group, some of the most committed and "expert" nursing mothers were those who had worked very hard to earn that designation.

For some women, nursing is not a comfortable activity at first and may actually be painful at times. If this is because the baby's latch is not right, the midwives will help you practise until you and the baby can do it by rote. If the baby is catching too little of your breast in the mouth when he or she sucks, the mouth will wear at the skin and tissue of your nipple. If you think your baby has not latched on correctly, take him off—no matter how long it took you to get him on. Your breasts are the tools you need to feed him, you must take good care of them.

Sore nipples often heal well if you expose them to air; try to skip the bra and the shirt, too, if possible. Nursing pads will keep your shirt dry, but they will also keep your nipples wet, and if they are sore this will exacerbate the problem. Expressing milk over any cracks in your skin will help the healing. There are many nipple creams on the market, but not all of them are good for your skin or O.K. for your baby. Your midwife will advise you on the best brands available.

If your breasts feel sore because they are engorged and you can't get the baby to relieve you, try expressing some milk after applying hot washcloths to them or taking a hot bath. Sometimes your milk ducts, which run all across your breasts and up under your armpit, can become blocked. Gentle massage, frequent nursing (in a variety of positions), and hot compresses can relieve this condition too. If a duct remains blocked for too long, it can lead to a condition called mastitis, which is an infection of the breast. Mastitis causes burning pain in the breast and is sometimes accompanied by a red line and a fever. If you suspect you have mastitis, consult your midwife, who will assess whether antibiotics are required.

### Euphoria and Baby Bliss

Some women report a sense of ecstatic joy following their son or daughter's birth. Sometimes this joy manifests itself as a great deal of energy.

Baby bliss is a great feeling. Enjoy it, but be careful not to overdo it. Though your emotions are upbeat, your body may need time to recover from its difficult job. Doing too much too soon could precipitate an emotional crash in a week or two. Unfortunately, this is often the time when the help you've arranged for after the birth—whether your partner's or of friends and family—is ending, as these people return to their regular routine of work and their own lives.

### Bonding

A lot has been written about the magical process of bonding with your baby. What does it mean, and are you doing it? Many parents feel that they have been so busy taking care of the practical stuff that they have had no time to bond. Just as everyone has a different birth story, parents all take different paths to discover their relationship with their babies. Some people say they looked at their babies and felt as if they had known them forever. Other people experience a slow discovery of their feelings for their children. One way or another, you and your baby are getting to know each other on a minute-by-minute basis. All that "basic" stuff you do is tying you to each other in ways that you may not realize for a long, long time. Whether it clicks right away, or you realize one day that you know just how your little guy likes to be bounced to sleep, the hard work you do in the early days is essential.

### Feeling Bad

If you are one of the people who do *not* experience euphoria at your child's arrival, don't be alarmed. Most parents of infants find it something of a struggle to deal with the reality of a baby's needs; mothers, in particular, are taxed with the physical demands on their bodies. On top of that, the same wild hormonal shifts that produce extreme emotional highs for some moms can produce lows for others.

It's important to let your midwives know how you feel, even if your mood fluctuates. They will talk you through some of your concerns and can reassure you about your emotional situation. Most "baby blues" are minor and pass quickly. If your negative feelings linger, the midwives can assist you in getting help so that you can ultimately be happy and enjoy your new son or daughter.

If ever you feel you or your baby are in danger because of your mood, discuss this immediately with your midwife or another health care practitioner. Postpartum depression can be very serious and can arise anytime within the first year after you have given birth. If you suspect you are experiencing a depression, get professional help for accurate diagnosis and the necessary treatment.

## Beyond You and Baby

### Do You Need Extra Help?

In Sheila Kitzinger's beautiful book *The Home Birth Book* she talks about the "babymoon": a time when your new family can enjoy one another without interruption or schedules and expectations, other than those imposed by your newborn.

When considering what kind of help you might need after your child is born, keep the babymoon in mind. If you invite relatives into your home, or hire assistance, will the additional people give you more time to relax with your baby or cause stress? Anyone who comes into your home in the early days should recognize the importance of your new family unit, and should understand that the best way to assist is by tending to the practical aspects of the house: food, laundry, answering the phone and so on. Much the same sorts of personality traits are required of a support person in the early days as were required during labour. You need someone who will support your choices, boost your confidence and leave when you tell him or her to go. In the first few weeks of a baby's life, you do not want to be playing hostess. You need to be catered to.

**Family support after the baby arrives**

I must admit that I was shocked by how I felt for the next week. It was still painful to sit down, and breastfeeding required so much sitting. I felt unprepared for this pain, having heard women talk only about the pain of childbirth, not afterwards. I was light-headed and dizzy and didn't even get out of bed for five days to make my own breakfast.

Instead I let my mother take care of us. She'd basically packed her bags the moment she'd gotten the call from my partner and driven seven hours straight to arrive at our door. She was fabulous. She cooked and cleaned and made herself useful. When she left after the five days, I cried for an hour, then got up and felt ready to be on my own.

—*Linda, mother of one, stepmother of two*

*Parental Relations*

Having a baby can challenge a relationship and strain both partners in their dealings with each other. But it can also bring people together as never before. It can even do both these things in the same relationship. It's important to recognize that your new roles make incredible demands on you both, especially if you're first-time parents. It's obvious that you need to be there for your baby, but you can do this best by caring for each other.

Your midwives can talk to you and your partner about how best to help you recover, depending on your needs, and ways that your partner can contribute most effectively. Sometimes a source of stress is that partners do not know how to help in a meaningful way. The mother and the baby are at the centre, and partners sometimes feel as though they are not needed or valued. The mother–baby relationship may be intense and may even seem exclusive. This can make it hard for others in the family, particularly partners. Couples, especially in families with many kids, have to find ways to care for everyone.

Once the first, difficult days are over, things will return to a (new) normal. This new normal will probably involve a constant shifting of roles and responsibilities as your baby grows. Just like the nursing, and the sleeping, it's all a fine balance that needs to be tested to get it just right. Soon the balance will adjust to meet changing circumstances.

### Introducing Your Baby

At some point, you will want to let go of the babymoon and introduce your child to a wider circle of friends and family. The timing should depend less on social expectations than on your health and feelings and your baby's personality. Miranda's first child was happy to attend every event going, from the time she was a week old—as long as it didn't involve more than a few minutes away from the breast. Miranda's second child was overstimulated by things that most adults and children wouldn't even notice, such as a TV on at low volume or shadows flickering across the couch behind her. So she had to be introduced to new situations more cautiously.

Keeping your plans flexible and manageable for your whole family is a good idea. If your first few engagements go smoothly, you'll be much more likely to keep trying for a social life with your baby. If you do too much, too quickly, a few bad experiences can turn you off for a long time.

If you must attend a social event early in your child's life, make sure there is somewhere quiet to rest, should either of you need to make an escape. People should be more than happy to accommodate your needs as a new mother, but if you are concerned about their reaction, warn them ahead of time that your visit will be brief, or that you will need to take a lot of breaks.

Some mothers and some babies are happy to let go and have the kid passed around to the relatives or the neighbours. If you or your baby feel uncomfortable in this situation, then prepare yourself ahead of time to say so, or arm yourself with an excuse, such as "My midwife thinks he has a little cold and suggests he not be handled," or some other slight lie that produces the desired result. You may not know how you will feel about people holding and touching your baby, and it bears some thought ahead of time.

*(Un)Helpful Advice*

Everybody knows about babies, because everybody was one. That's the sarcastic comment Miranda's husband uses to combat unwanted help from people who aren't his children's parents, but think they could do it better. Even the most seasoned mother or grandfather is at a disadvantage when it comes to your kid, because she's *your* kid! You are the authority.

### Opposition to breastfeeding

I had more negative comments about breastfeeding than I did about having the baby at home. My son was tongue-tied (when the tongue is attached too tightly to the mouth), and they all said, "Why are you putting yourself through that?" or "Why don't you just give him a bottle?" instead of saying "Let's find somebody who can help you with that."

*—Janine, mother of two*

That's not to say that people do not have ideas for tricks and techniques that might work for you. The things that we have learned about parenting were best gleaned from others' examples, combined with trial and error. Only you can separate the useful advice from the superfluous or bossy. Just remember that the best way to parent your baby is to pay attention to the signals that he or she gives you and then respond.

This book is all about advice and information. Midwives are all about information and support. But you are the expert on your own family, your role in it and your child.

### Helping a mother find her own answers

When I went to the six-week visit at the midwives, that day he was crying and crying, and I felt incompetent. I kept saying, "Is this the way you hold him?" almost exaggerating that I had no idea how to do it. I felt embarrassed almost that he was hollering. I felt like at six weeks I should be acting a little more in control. The midwife was so great. She would say, "What do you think? How do you think you should hold him?" In my experience, any emotional reassurances they made would eventually come from myself. They helped the answers come from me. It was amazing.

—Jessica, mother of two

## Things to Look For in a Newborn

To ensure that your baby is thriving, the midwives will monitor his or her progress by observing certain indicators each time they see you. First they will make sure the baby is taking in enough nourishment. You and your midwives will have many discussions about how the baby nurses: how long, how frequently and the quality of the latch. The midwife will also help you assess your child's well-being by showing you how to inspect diapers for amount and quality of urine, as well as indications of bowel movements. As mentioned earlier in this chapter, newborn stool goes from black and tar-like to yellow and mustardy. Sometimes in the early days you may also find a bit of orange or red dust-like substance in the diaper. This is not a cause for concern and should clear up within a few days. Newborn girls also occasionally discharge a bit of blood or mucous from their vaginas. Boys and girls can have swollen breasts or excrete a milky substance from their breasts in response to all the hormones they received from their mothers. Again, this is temporary and will clear up within a day or two. When your midwife checks in next, mention any of these variations to her, so she can note them.

Another all-important way to make sure your baby is getting enough nourishment is to keep track of his weight. Midwives carry newborn scales that have fabric slings in which your baby rests while being weighed. Many babies sleep through this procedure, which is a regular and frequent part of newborn checkups. Babies usually lose some weight after birth and gain it back within a few days. This loss followed by continuous gain is a solid indicator that your baby is healthy and thriving.

Checking your baby's temperature is something your midwives will do every time they see you. An elevated temperature (normal infant temperature is between 36.5° C and 37.5° C under the arm) is very dangerous in a little baby and can indicate a problem. A fever in a newborn baby is always treated very seriously. Having a good quality thermometer on hand is therefore a good idea.

Sometimes babies pick up the mother's naturally occurring yeast as they move through the birth canal. Called thrush, this is a common culprit for recurrent breastfeeding problems. If a baby's body absorbs the yeast, it can make the inside of her mouth irritated and painful so that nursing becomes difficult. It can also cause painful diaper rashes in the infant that won't go away. The yeast can be passed back to the mother, making her breasts sore and painful when nursing. If your baby has problems nursing, look for signs of thrush. White patches on the inside of his or her mouth that won't wipe off and a bright red diaper rash are symptoms that you can ask your midwife about. A mother might experience shooting pain deep in her breast when nursing. Outward signs are small red or white patches on the breast and reddish or purple nipples. Both you and the baby could experience one or all of these symptoms. Possible treatments include painting gentian violet (available in drugstores) on your breasts and your baby's diaper area or using anti-fungal cream available by prescription. You will need to air out your breasts and frequently change your bras, nursing pads and shirts, since the yeast attaches itself effectively to clothes. Wash clothes carefully in very hot water. Ask your midwife about other available treatments.

Babies need to feed frequently, and they need sleep. Their parents also need them to sleep so that they can get rest. But babies should not go too long without feeding, especially in the first few days of life. If you have a baby who is a real sleeper, you may need to regularly rouse him or her for feedings. After the baby's feeding pattern and weight gain is established, you can take a more relaxed approach, knowing your baby will wake when he or she needs to be fed.

If your normally alert baby is lethargic and difficult to rouse, call your midwife immediately. An overly jittery baby may also be in need of a checkover. Of course, for a new parent, it may be difficult to judge these situations. Your midwives will combine their skill in newborn assessment with your knowledge of your baby to decide whether he or she needs medical assistance. Should your child require more help, the midwives will make sure you receive attention from the appropriate professional. Most often, though, your midwives will perform the wonderful service of addressing your concerns, making the all-important checks and then reassuring you that your baby is just fine.

## ◈ If You Want to Read More . . .

*Bestfeeding: Getting Breastfeeding Right for You*, by Mary Renfrew, Chloe Fisher and Suzanne Arms (Berkeley, California: Celestial Arts, 2000).

*Dr. Jack Newman's Guide to Breastfeeding*, by Jack Newman and Teresa Pitman (Toronto: HarperCollins, 2000).

*What to Expect When You're Expecting*, by Arlene Eisenberg, Heidi E. Murkoff and Sandee E. Hathaway (New York: Workman Publishing, Inc., 1991).

*Wise Woman Herbal for the Childbearing Year*, by Susun S. Weed (Woodstock, New York: Ash Tree Publishing, 1986).

*The Womanly Art of Breastfeeding*, by Gwen Gotsch and Judy Torgar (Schaumberg, Illinois: La Leche League International, 1991).

*Your Baby and Child: From Birth to Age Five* (2nd ed.), by Penelope Leach (New York: Alfred A. Knopf, 1995).

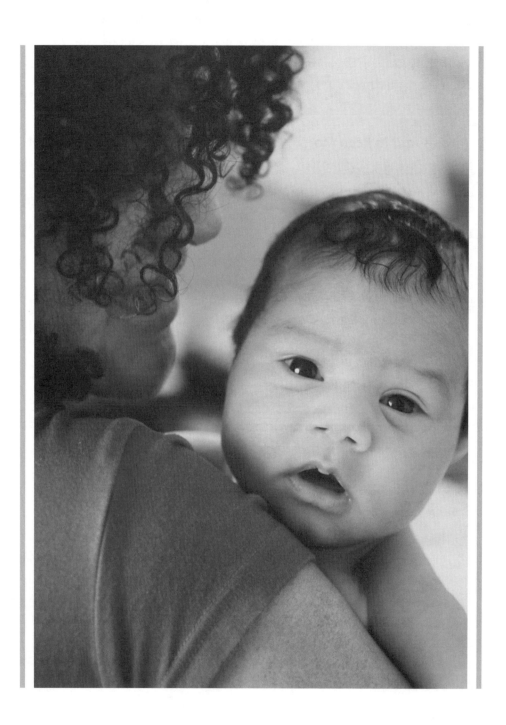

## Twelve

# Saying Goodbye, Staying Connected

When helping to organize a reunion for past clients of our Toronto practice, Miranda encountered a woman whose birth seemed like it had happened yesterday. "It's so funny that you called right now," she said. "I was just thinking of my midwives. Today is my daughter's ninth birthday!"

Whether you ever forget the pain of childbirth is a subject of debate for mothers and grandmothers everywhere. But most women do remember their caregivers' participation in the birth, or lack thereof. If a woman is unhappy about the support she received, that feeling will surface when she recalls her child's arrival. If she feels that her caregivers were there for her, their presence remains a vital part of the experience.

### The Final Visit

At about six weeks after your baby's birth, you will probably have a final visit with your midwives. Most mothers will come to the midwives' office for this visit. The midwives will weigh your baby and inquire whether you are still bleeding and, if so, how much. They will also ask you for a progress report on the baby's feeding and sleeping, and, as always, find out how you are feeling.

At this visit you may also have a conversation about birth control options. Your midwife may suggest you see your family doctor at some point in the near future, perhaps to arrange for birth control. You might also talk about nutrition and changes that your body is going through. You may also get a copy of some parts of your chart to keep and share with your doctor. This will provide helpful information about what tests you received, what the results were, and how your birth went.

Finally, if you have no lingering concerns of a serious nature, the midwives will officially sign off on your chart and discharge you.

Most mothers, and some fathers too, note that this transition feels abrupt, no matter how buffered it is with hugs and invitations to keep in touch. The midwives have seen you through an intense and important time in your life, but now it's time to move on. Suddenly you remember that midwives are professionals—committed professionals, but professionals nonetheless.

Midwives in busy practices may be involved in caring for more than 80 women a year, on the same 24-hour basis they offered you. In the course of a career, a midwife may be present at hundreds, perhaps thousands of births. Midwives everywhere are asked, "What will happen when I don't see you any more?"

### Moving out of the midwives' care

As I anticipate another birth, I find myself also looking ahead even farther, to six weeks postpartum. I fully expect to be sad to leave midwifery care. It is like losing a friend. One friend even told me that she toyed with having another baby just so that she could be in midwifery care again! It also spoils you for any other health care. I appreciate my doctor's care very much, and we see him fairly frequently for various childhood ailments. But it simply does not compare with the warmth, respect and normalcy I've come to value from midwives. If only other practitioners could follow their lead.

—*Rebecca, mother of three*

Midwives and midwifery clients have ways of keeping a relationship going. Bringing the baby by for periodic weigh-ins and to show him or her off is always popular, and you can ask your midwife about doing this. Some parents keep their midwives updated with cards, sent on the anniversary of their baby's birth, which include pictures of the child. Others find ways to become involved in midwifery advocacy, which keeps them connected with the community. Whatever you choose, your relationship with your midwives will be necessarily different than it was when you were in their care.

A midwife in Alberta reports getting calls from women looking for advice about everything from when to start feeding their children solid food to interpreting fevers. In some places where physicians are unavailable, midwives advocate taking on more aspects of "well-woman care," like writing prescriptions for birth control pills and doing pap smears.

Some practices maintain connections with their clients by offering postpartum support groups for mothers of new babies. Others host "birth circles," where mothers and expectant mothers come to discuss the birth process. If there a group like this does not exist at your practice, you could consider starting.

## Recalling Your Birth Experience

**Thinking back on the birth**

After the baby is born and the midwives come to your house, your focus remains on the baby. But going over what happened can continue on for months. It would be great to have some sort of support group in which that could happen.

—*Anne, mother of two*

Birth is a very intense time. Some women remember the births of their children with a vivid intensity, while others have trouble remembering the details, having gone through the actual experience in a fog. As you recall the events that took place during your birth, it can help to have those who were present compare notes. Your personal support people can tell their stories, and your midwives will be able to fill in other blanks for you. Some women find it very helpful to talk about the birth itself at the postpartum visits. When Sarah's first baby was born after an uneventful labour suddenly became serious in the final moments, the baby needed CPR and oxygen. Time seemed to stand still while her midwife and obstetrician (who also had pediatric training) worked on the baby. When the baby cried and someone said, "She is going to be fine," Sarah and her partner were finally able to rejoice in the birth of their daughter. But the next few hours were confusing and disorienting as tiredness set in and the baby could not be roused to nurse. They were able to go home very soon after the birth, but it wasn't until much later that Sarah understood the danger her baby had been in. In the weeks following the birth, Sarah had to ask her midwife, partner and sister what they remembered so that she could understand the events herself. Eventually, it dawned on her that she owed her baby's life, literally, to her midwife and obstetrician. As the years have passed and Sarah's daughter has grown, so has the significance of her birth story.

In some ways, the birth story is a combination of what you remember and what others tell you they recall. You will not be able to choose each moment of the labour and birth to become part of the story, so what moments will you choose? The significance of choosing, consciously or not, to remember some parts and not others will only appear much later in your child's life. Every birth experience has its highs and lows. Almost every woman feels there were times when she could not go on, or felt that she was the strongest, most powerful creature ever to walk the Earth. What will you remember?

Birth is a personal experience for everyone who takes part. Just because two people attend the same birth does not mean that their perception of it will be the same, or that they will tell the same story. Here is a father's take and a mother's take on the birth of their first daughter.

### Téa's birth (Daddy's version)

At 4:14 A.M. Brandie got up. I looked over and asked, "Are you O.K.?" In the dark, she looked over and replied, "I think my water broke." "You think?" I queried. Of course I was kind of expecting this, but how could she not know? I decided to see what she was thinking. "Do you think I should go to work today?" I said, knowing full well that today is the day and there is no way in hell I'm going to work. "Maybe," she answered. I, of course, was completely befuddled.

So Brandie went to the bathroom and checked: her water had broken for sure, and she had begun to have mild contractions. I always look on the positive side. I'd been saying for the last nine months that she was going to have a really easy labour, but she was always telling me how tough it would be. But these contractions were so mild, it was scary: 20 to 30 seconds every five to seven minutes.

We decided to get a couple of things done, get a quick bite of food, and prepare ourselves for the day. Again, I wanted to see where she was at. I asked, "So, what do you think? Should I get ready for work?" "Maybe," she said. I couldn't believe it! Then I knew she was in complete denial.

We called the midwives to tell them that Brandie was in labour and that she was having contractions but they were really light and easy. They said no problem, and to call them back when things began to get serious.

We went back to bed and watched a movie until 7:30 A.M., when Brandie decided the contractions were getting stronger; by my watch the contractions were 30 to 40 seconds, every two to three minutes. We got up. Brandie decided to try labouring sitting on the toilet while I paged the midwives. The midwife called us back at 8:00 A.M. We talked and she told us she'd get ready and come over.

Then Brandie's mood changed and she got quite serious about the process. We tried a couple of positions in the bathtub, but she felt more comfortable on the toilet, so we eventually moved back there. Brandie's mother came over, and we all hung out in the bathroom, taking the contractions one step at a time. I looked through our books and prenatal class workbook, but I couldn't find anywhere where they say the contractions can be as short as 30 seconds. All I could think was, Are we in serious labour or is this just early stuff?

When the midwife finally arrived, she did a quick examination of Brandie and said that she was at four centimetres. I was really hoping we'd gotten somewhere. Our midwife said we had to try some more positions. So we got up and slowly walked down the stairs. Brandie sat on a stepstool in the kitchen for about 15 minutes, then we slowly made our way back up the stairs. We proceeded to the bathroom, where Brandie tried getting down on all fours. That lasted only one contraction. Wow! She said that made it hurt way more and quickly decided to sit back on the toilet.

Suddenly, Brandie's mood changed, and she said that she was starting to push! Oh my. I called to our midwife downstairs, "She's starting to push!"

We got Brandie to the bed, and the midwife started to give her an exam, but it was evident the baby was coming soon. I glanced at the clock, and it was just after 11:00 A.M. Wow that was fast! Brandie gave another push and we could see the top of the head! Oh my! The midwife got Brandie's mom to grab a bowl of hot water and toss some washcloths into it, to use for hot compresses. The midwife told her to drop the bottle of almond oil into the bowl to heat it up. About 15 seconds after that, the midwife asked for the almond oil. Brandie's mom got the cap off the warmed bottle, but at that moment Brandie had one more contraction, and whoooosh! Baby girl Téa Alexandria Susanna Serack was born! That was at 11:09 A.M. Holy cow!

—*Garrett, father of one*

### Téa's birth (Mommy's version)

On Thursday, February 21st, I noticed some bloody streaks on my panties and discovered that my mucous plug was coming out. I got very excited as I knew then that labour was getting near. I called Garrett and told him what was happening, saying, "I just thought you should know." He didn't know how to take it, but it certainly distracted him and made it hard for him to concentrate on work! I looked in my pregnancy book, and it said that most women who have a "bloody show" go into labour within three days.

At my midwife's appointment that day, my midwife reviewed with me what I should expect and when I to call should I start going into labour. Later that night I noticed that the mucous had changed and now I was actually spotting some darker blood. I put on a pad. Although I was excited, I certainly still didn't think that I was going to go into labour as early as the next morning!

At 3:00 A.M., I woke up and had to go to the bathroom. I went back to bed, feeling a few minor cramps but nothing that seemed significant. An hour later after lying there trying to get back to sleep, I had this gushing feeling. So I sat right up and got out of bed. Garrett woke up with a start, and I told him, "I think my water broke." He got up in a real hurry!

I think I probably sat down and started to feel a contraction. So we turned on the TV and sat through a couple of contractions, but they were only 30 seconds long, and were about five to seven minutes apart, and not very painful. We got up to take a shower. Garrett brought out the video camera at about 5:30 A.M., and we taped a little bit of my "first" experiences. We watched a bit of television. Then Garrett made some fruit shakes, just to make sure I ate something to keep my energy up while I still could eat. We then put on a movie and watched that for a bit. I was finding that when the contractions came (they were now two minutes apart but still only 30 seconds long) I didn't know what to do with my hands. The contractions were getting harder to take while lying on the bed. I decided to get up. I remembered that my yoga instructor had commented that the toilet felt like a good place to labour. So that was the first place I went. Sure enough, it made it a lot easier, especially when I would gush more amniotic fluid now and again.

At 6:30 A.M. we called my mom and she arrived at my house by 8:00 A.M. Garrett kept asking when to call the midwives. He looked in our Bradley Method book to see what "stage" we were at, but there was no mention of contractions that were 30 seconds long and two minutes apart. Since my mother was already there, I figured we didn't need the midwives to come over yet. Still, I thought we should probably call them and let them know I had started labour and that today would be the day. The midwife on call for the day told me to have a bath, and that she would have some breakfast and a shower and then make her way over.

I was amazed at how conversational I was between contractions, and how I felt absolutely no pain in between them. I had to moan and close my eyes during the contractions, though. I told Garrett to run me a bath. When I got in, it felt O.K. It was hard at first to figure out how best to get comfortable during contractions in this new environment. I only tried two positions: one involved just sitting normally, the other, kneeling and hanging over the side of the tub. At one point, I actually got a four-minute reprieve. The contractions came back much stronger, so I decided I wanted to sit on the toilet again.

Just before 10:00 A.M., I was thinking, "O.K., I am about ready for this to be over already!" I was also thinking, "How long does it take a midwife to have breakfast and a shower? Where is she?" Once she finally arrived, she got me to lie down on the bed so she could check my dilation—that was very uncomfortable. I did not like having a contraction and trying to lie down at the same time. I felt out of control. She got me in a good position, checked me, and told us that we were only at four centimetres, but that it was good and that she could feel the baby's head. I was pretty disheartened that I had a lot of work ahead of me still. Garrett admitted to me later that he too felt discouraged.

My midwife suggested that we get up and move around, which I wasn't so keen on doing by this time. But she said we needed to get things going and get the baby in the right position. We got out the exercise/birthing ball, and I sat on it for a while. Then the midwife had me get up and walk. We made it down the stairs, although halfway down I had another contraction. We went into the kitchen. I leaned over the eating bar, and she told me to spread my legs and to rock my bum, so I did that twice.

Garrett grabbed a strawberry Popsicle for me and tried to feed it to me. The first time was fine, but then it started to drip, so I irritably told him to put it in a cup. Then he tried to feed it to me again. It was still dripping, so I tried to tell him to feed it to me over the cup. When he didn't understand, I grabbed it from him and fed myself.

My midwife had me sit on a low stool and she supported me from behind. After two tough contractions in this position, she showed Garrett how to support me. After a while the contractions felt a bit more under control. She told me that if things were getting too comfortable in any one position, then I should change it.

So I decided after a bit that I wanted to go back upstairs to try the ball again. I got on the ball, and then decided that I should try on my hands and knees. When the next contraction came, I felt terrified. At first there was the pain of the contraction, then I felt like I wanted to poop, and then this overwhelming sensation hit me. It was very painful, and I started to scream. I half got up and didn't know what to do. I sat down on the toilet and instantly felt the same thing. My instinct was to close my legs. Then I realized that my body was trying to push the baby out. I yelled at Garrett that I had to push! He got a bit panicky and ran to tell our midwife.

My midwife ran upstairs and told me that we needed to get me off the toilet. My legs were shaking violently, I felt very weak, very terrified and very out of control. When the pushing started to happen again, I didn't know what to do with myself. I screamed to Garrett that I didn't think I could do this, but I was mostly referring to getting off the toilet and walking all the way over to the bed. It seemed to me so far away. My midwife convinced me that as soon as the urge to push was over, we had to do it. So we did. The whole way to the bed I was saying, "Hurry, hurry!" because I didn't know when my body would push again. I barely got on the bed and again screamed as my uterus pushed and the pain from the perineum overwhelmed me. My midwife told me I had to listen to her, that I had to push slowly. I remember one push where she had me touch the top of my baby's head. It felt soft and squishy and slimy, not at all like a head. Then the push started and my midwife kept telling me, "Slowly, slowly." I was thinking, "Yeah, right. Like I have any control over this." But at the beginning of the last push, I did feel a bit calmer and tried to slow the pushes down. However, before I knew it, the pain intensified around the perineum, and then the baby's head appeared and, seconds later, the baby was born. I remember the midwife telling me to lift my shirt, and she placed the baby on top of my belly. I remember seeing this wide-eyed blue creature, who was crying. My midwife put a towel over both of us to keep us warm and asked me what the sex was. It had been a couple of minutes and I hadn't even thought to check! I lifted the baby up and saw her swollen genitals. But I was too dazed to figure out if that was really a girl or if it was actually a boy. Garrett said, "It's a girl!" I was truly amazed.

—*Brandie, mother of one*

One approach to creating the story of your child's birth is to write down your recollections at intervals in the days afterward. Don't read over what you have written yet. Just make notes as you remember things. You might want to have your partner or other participants write down their impressions too. Much later, once the event is no longer fresh and the story has been told out loud many times, looking back at what you have written can be fascinating. Over time, your birth story will become distilled. Your child may want to hear this version of the story again and again. In the end, it belongs to him or her.

Often, a mother's feelings about herself and the birth take time to develop. Some midwifery practices have devised ways to connect mothers before and after birth. For example, they may have prenatal groups, postpartum groups, birth circles and buddy systems. If your practice does not offer these services, you can ask your midwife to put you in touch with other clients who may have children the same age as yours or who have had similar birth experiences.

## The Midwifery Legacy

One of the most telling and interesting things that women bring up about midwifery care is the lasting effect it has had on them as people and as parents. For most women, ourselves included, this "midwifery legacy" is a complete surprise; it's an unexpected and wonderful by-product of our care.

At first, the number of decisions you must make about your pregnancy and birth may seem daunting. The thought has occurred to many midwifery clients that it would be easier if the midwives just made the decisions for them. In the end, though, the planning and thought required of a midwifery client helps prepare a woman for parenting, where decision-making and advocacy are required many times a day. As a midwifery client you are the ultimate authority. You realize it's your body and your baby. This realization, combined with the great support midwives provide during the really difficult tasks of birth and in the early days with a newborn, helps many women conclude that ultimately they can do anything.

**Building a mother's confidence**

They did all the right things. They gave me the message that I knew what to do. The key was to listen to myself and my baby. They led me to believe in myself and helped me become the mother I now am.

*—Diane, mother of one*

## Finding a Physician

Midwives care for their clients—both mothers and babies—for about six weeks after the birth. If you already have a family doctor, returning to his or her care with your baby may go smoothly. But if you have had sporadic personal health care prior to pregnancy, when you leave the care of the midwives you may want to find a doctor who can give you and your child more attention.

Family doctors are generalists by training but are specialists in your overall care. Their mandate is to take an overall approach to your health and well-being and to act as the conduit to more specialized care should you need it. If you have or find a family doctor with whom you feel comfortable, he or she may also be an excellent caregiver for your infant; theoretically, this person can continue to provide care for your child into adulthood.

Some families actively seek out a pediatrician to care for their child in the first years of life. The advantage of pediatricians is that they specialize in childhood ailments and conditions. However, pediatricians are not familiar with your *entire* family's health. Sometimes it can be hard to book an appointment with them on short notice because, in addition to their regular patients, they receive referrals from family doctors.

When approaching any new health care provider, whether a family doctor or a specialist, you will want to know how you can get assistance on short notice and at odd hours. Does the doctor have an on-call service with other members of a practice group, or have privileges at a hospital with a 24-hour clinic?

In many places, doctors are very difficult to find. Even in urban centres, many doctors are no longer taking new patients; in smaller places, such as remote or rural communities, there may be only one choice. If you find yourself in a situation where a certain doctor is the only one available and you feel ambivalent about that doctor, then you will definitely have to advocate for the kind of care you want.

In medical care, as in midwifery care, you have a right to know your options. If you are seeing a doctor, you can still ask questions, challenge assumptions and continue to be informed about your own care and your child's. Know what you are entitled to and ask for the information that will help you make the right decision for you and your baby.

Medical procedures and decisions cannot be carried out or made without your consent. This applies to everything from vaccinations to more serious operations. What is right for you and your child may not be the same as what is right for your friend's or neighbour's family, and your doctor needs to recognize your ultimate authority.

## Providing Feedback to Your Midwives

Some midwifery practices offer a formal, anonymous mechanism for providing feedback through a written evaluation form. Filling out forms is probably the last thing you want to do as the parent of a new baby. However, your participation is extremely important to maintaining and improving the quality of midwifery care. Think over your care and consider in what ways it met your needs, exceeded them or fell below them. These impressions are vitally important if midwives are to remain woman-centred and responsive to their clients.

Of course, it may be difficult to provide constructive criticism if you are concerned about offending a person, especially one who has had such a tremendous impact on your life. If your practice does not offer an anonymous mechanism for providing feedback, you may want to suggest it. Other suggestions from mothers and midwifery clients include providing your midwives with a written birth story (including all its highs and lows), or writing a goodbye letter in order to leave your midwives with a record of your thoughts about the birth experience and the care you received.

If you have serious concerns or complaints about the quality of your care and have failed to get an appropriate response from your midwives about them, you can make a complaint to the college of midwives in your area. The college is a professional body that governs the conduct and standards of midwives practising in a legislated province or territory.

## Staying Connected to Midwifery

Many families wonder what they can do to show their appreciation for the support midwives provide for almost a year. Some families try to reciprocate by lobbying on behalf of the midwifery profession and attempting to extend the midwifery option to more women.

Midwifery consumer strength is high in provinces where legislation is pending or where funding issues remain outstanding. In Alberta, where midwives are legislated but not funded, midwifery consumers publish two magazines to get the word out about the kind of care midwives provide. Nova Scotia has a support group called the Midwifery Coalition of Nova Scotia, which has been advocating for legislated, funded midwifery for more than 20 years.

Opportunities exist for supporting midwifery on a large or local scale. In southern Ontario a group called MABEL (Midwife-Assisted Birth Education League) works to provide information to the public about what midwives stand for and the work they do. Its outreach has included a calendar on the theme of breastfeeding and a book of birth stories. The group also sets up information tables staffed by members, at local malls.

Informal reunions, such as the picnic our practice hosts in a local park in late spring, give past clients the opportunity to stay in contact with their midwives and keep midwifery grounded in the community. Those reunions take considerable time to organize—something that the harried midwives are usually unable to accomplish. When past or present clients take on this role, then midwives can get re-acquainted with former clients.

Another way to remain connected with midwifery is to sit on advisory committees or task forces or to become involved in advocating for midwifery within government funding agencies and on boards of midwifery education programs. Midwifery journals and professional midwifery associations also value consumer voices.

### Making the transition from midwifery care

My first midwife dropped by each day for the first few days after the birth to check on us. She tracked my recovery, weighed and checked Alec, and answered any concerns I had. The value of these home visits was priceless. I really appreciated being able to stay in our safe little cocoon world. When the final appointment with the midwives came, I was shaken. It was difficult to let go of their empathetic attention. Who would answer the many questions I had every day about my newborn? Having a child confirmed for me the vital need for community support around mothers and their families, which midwives, as skilled practitioners and wise caregivers, provide.

—*Erica, mother of one*

## Branching Out

Giving up that close relationship with a midwife is difficult for many people, but linking into a whole new network of parents your child's age can offset the feeling of loss and provide a great new beginning.

As we mentioned earlier, postpartum groups and birthing circles are perfect places to find new allies. Groups such as La Leche League also operate in many parts of the country, offering support for breastfeeding and mothering.

In fact, parenting friends are so important that long before Miranda's kids were looking for playmates of their own, Miranda was trolling the neighbourhoods trying to find new playmates for herself. Having friends who have little kids who are nursing, then toilet training, then entering school at the same time as yours allows for a certain kind of sympathy that no one else can provide. Oh, people can say they remember the sleepless times, but nothing beats hearing from other parents who were up for the same four hours you were last night!

Of course, among the things mothers and fathers of young children talk about is the birth experience. It used to be that a family that had chosen midwifery would know most of the other families in the area that had made the same choice. But as midwifery extends its reach, more and more midwifery clients are finding that they meet new people who have had their own birth experience with midwives. As well, part of the reason that mothers choose midwifery in the first place is that they heard about it from a sister, a friend, a colleague or a parent in the park.

If this was your introduction to midwifery, then you can pass your experience and enthusiasm along to another parent.


## Why Midwifery?

When we did the research for this book, midwives across the country told us that one of their primary motivations for becoming midwives was to help women gain confidence in themselves through their births. Mothers who have managed to have a drug-free homebirth and those who have had C-sections after many hours of labour can both come away feeling empowered. The business of babies is an emotional one, filled with health and social concerns. Midwives devote themselves to accompanying women and their families as they begin this incredible journey into parenthood.

## ◈ If You Want to Read More . . .

*What to Expect the First Year*, by Arlene Eisenberg, Heidi E. Murkoff and Sandee E. Hathaway (New York: Workman Publishing, Inc., 1996).

*Your Baby and Child: From Birth to Age Five* (2nd ed.), by Penelope Leach (New York: Alfred A. Knopf, 1995).

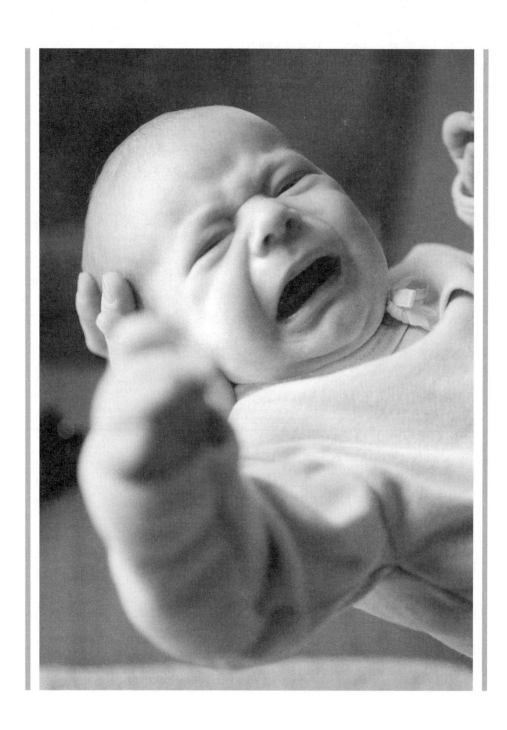

# Bibliography

Arms, Suzanne. *Immaculate Deception II: Myth Magic and Birth*. Berkeley, California: Celestial Arts, 1994.

Barrett, Joyce and Teresa Pitman. *Pregnancy and Birth: The Best Evidence*. Toronto: Key Porter Books, 1999.

Barrington, Eleanor. *Midwifery Is Catching*. Toronto: NC Press Limited, 1985.

Bradley, Robert A. *Husband-Coached Childbirth*. Sherman Oaks, California: Bantam, 1996.

Burtch, Brian. *Trials of Labour: The Re-emergence of Midwifery*. Montreal and Kingston: McGill-Queen's University Press, 1994.

Campion, Mukti Jain. *The Baby Challenge: A Handbook on Pregnancy for Women with a Physical Disability*. London: Routledge, 1990.

Canadian Association of Midwives. *Canadian Journal of Midwifery Research and Practice*.

Curtis, Glade B. *Your Pregnancy Week-by-Week*. Tucson, Arizona: Fisher Books, 1994.

Devries, Raymond (et al.). *Birth by Design: Pregnancy, Maternity Care, and Midwifery in North America and Europe*. New York: Routledge, 2001.

Douglas, Ann. *The Mother of All Pregnancy Books: An All-Canadian Guide to Conception, Birth & Everything in Between*. Toronto: CDG Books, 2000.

Douglas, Ann. *Trying Again: A Guide to Pregnancy After Miscarriage, Stillbirth and Infant Loss*. Toronto: Taylor Publishing, 2000.

Ehrenreich, Barbara and Deirdre English. *Witches, Midwives, and Nurses: A History of Women Healers*. New York: The Feminist Press, 1973.

Eisenberg, Arlene, Heidi E. Murkoff and Sandee E. Hathaway. *What to Expect the First Year*. New York: Workman Publishing, Inc., 1996.

Eisenberg, Arlene, Heidi E. Murkoff and Sandee E. Hathaway. *What to Expect When You're Expecting*. New York: Workman Publishing, Inc., 1991.

England, Pam and Rob Horowitz. *Birthing from Within: An Extra-Ordinary Guide to Childbirth Preparation*. Albuquerque, New Mexico: Partera Press, 1998.

Gaskin, Ina May. *Spiritual Midwifery* (3rd ed.). Summertown, Tennessee: The Book Publishing Company, 1990.

Gotsch, Gwen and Judy Torgar. *The Womanly Art of Breastfeeding*. Schaumberg, Illinois: La Leche League International, 1991.

Hunsburger, Winifred Wallace. *One Mother to Another*. Saskatoon, Saskatchewan: Fifth House Publishers, 1992.

Kitzinger, Sheila. *The Complete Book of Pregnancy and Childbirth* (new ed.). London: Dorling Kindersley Limited, 1996.

Kitzinger, Sheila. *The Experience of Childbirth* (5th ed.). Harmondsworth: Penguin, 1987.

Kitzinger, Sheila. *Homebirth: The Essential Guide to Giving Birth Outside of the Hospital*. London: Dorling Kindersley Limited, 1991. Reissued in 2001 by Dorling Kindersley Limited as *Birth Your Way: Choosing Birth at Home or in a Birth Centre*.

Kitzinger, Sheila (ed.). *The Midwife Challenge* (new ed.). London: Pandora Press, 1991.

Leach, Penelope. *Your Baby and Child: From Birth to Age Five* (2nd ed.). New York: Alfred A. Knopf, 1995.

Leboyer, Frederick. *Birth Without Violence: Revised Edition of the Classic*. Rochester, Vermont: Inner Traditions International, 2002.

Newman, Jack and Teresa Pitman. *Dr. Jack Newman's Guide to Breastfeeding*. Toronto: HarperCollins, 2000.

Odent, Dr. Michael. *Birth Reborn*. New York: Random House, 1984.

Renfrew, Mary, Chloe Fisher and Suzanne Arms. *Bestfeeding: Getting Breastfeeding Right For You*. Berkeley, California: Celestial Arts, 2000.

Rothman, Barbara Katz. *The Encyclopedia of Childbearing*. New York: Henry Holt and Company, 1993.

Rothman, Barbara Katz. *In Labor: Women and Power in the Birthplace*. New York: Norton, 1991.

Sears, William and Martha Sears. *The Birth Book*. Boston: Little, Brown and Company, 1994.

Shroff, Farah M. (ed.). *The New Midwifery: Reflections on Renaissance and Regulation*. Toronto: Women's Press, 1997.

Simkin, Penny. *The Birth Partner*. Boston: The Harvard Common Press, 1989.

The Society of Obstetricians and Gynecologists of Canada. *Healthy Beginnings: Your Handbook for Pregnancy and Birth* (2nd ed.). Ottawa: The Society of Obstetricians and Gynecologists of Canada, 2000.

Weed, Susun S. *Wise Woman Herbal for the Childbearing Year*. Woodstock, New York: Ash Tree Publishing, 1986.

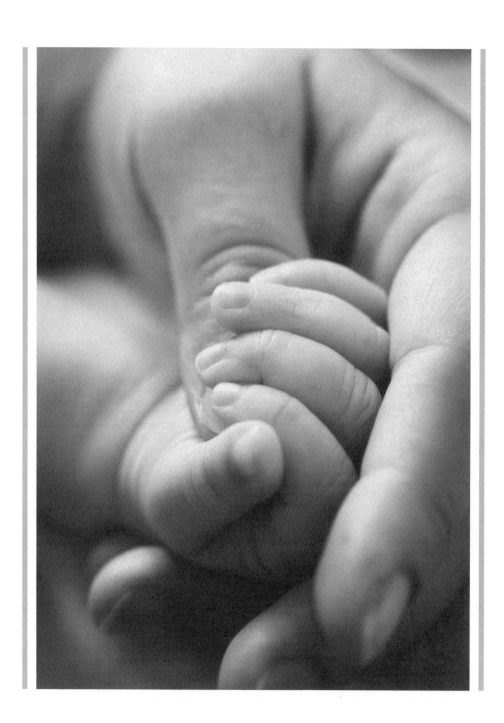

# Appendix

## Professional Associations

Canadian Association of Midwives
Web www.canadianmidwives.org
Email admin@canadianmidwives.org

### Alberta
Alberta Association of Midwives
Main Post Office, Box 11957
Edmonton, AB
T5J 3L1
Tel (780) 425-5464
Web www.albertamidwives.com
Email albertamidwives@shaw.ca

### British Columbia
Midwives Association of British Columbia
#336 – 5740 Cambie Street
Vancouver, BC
V5Z 3A6
Tel (604) 736-5976
Fax (604) 736-5957
Web www.bcmidwives.com
Email mabc@telus.net

### Manitoba
Midwives Association of Manitoba
LL – 691 Wolseley Avenue
Winnipeg, MB
R3G 1C3
Tel (204) 788-8141
Fax (204) 772-6035
Web www.manitobamidwives.com
Email info@manitobamidwives.com

### Newfoundland and Labrador
Association of Midwives of Newfoundland and
   Labrador
c/o Labrador Health Centre
Station A, HVGB
NF & LB
A0P 1E0
Tel (709) 897-2000 x 2210
Fax (709) 777-7037
Web www.ucs.mun.ca/~pherbert

*Nova Scotia*
Association of Nova Scotia Midwives
PO Box 968
Wolfville, NS
B0P IX0
Tel (902) 582-7133

*New Brunswick*
Midwives Association of New Brunswick/
    Association des sages femmes du Nouveau
    Brunswick
104 Bessborough
Moncton, NB
EIE IP9
Tel (506) 389-9473
Web www.manb-asfnb.ca
Email midwives@manb-asfnb.ca

*Northwest Territories*
Midwives Association of the Northwest
    Territories and Nunavut
Box 995
Fort Smith, NWT
X0E 0P0
Tel (867) 872-7133
Email midwives.nwt.nu@auroranet.nt.ca
gbecker@auroranet.nt.ca

*Nunavut*
Midwives Association of the Northwest
    Territories and Nunavut
Rankin Inlet Birthing Centre
Postal Bag 298
Rankin Inlet, NU
X0C 0G0
Tel (867) 645-3961
Fax (867) 645-3940
Email midwives.nwt.nu@auroranet.nt.ca
gbecker@auroranet.nt.ca

*Ontario*
Association of Ontario Midwives
789 Don Mills Road, Suite 201
Toronto, ON
M3C IT5
Tel (416) 425-9974
Fax (416) 425-6905
Web www.aom.on.ca
Email admin@aom.on.ca

*Prince Edward Island*
Prince Edward Island Midwives Association
34 Russet Drive
Charlottetown, PEI
CIE IB7
Tel (902) 566-2135
Email mabel.england@pei.sympatico.ca

*Quebec*
Regroupment des Sages-Femmes du Québec
BP 354, succursale Côte-des-Neiges
Montréal, PQ
H3S 2S6
Tel (514) 738-8090
Fax (514) 738-0370
Email sages.femmes.qc@sympatico.ca

*Saskatchewan*
Midwives Association of Saskatchewan
2836 Angus Street
Regina, SK
S4S IN8
Tel (306) 586-2241
Fax (306) 522-0818
Email mackenziep@skyway.usask.ca

*Yukon*
Yukon Midwives
303 Hoge Street
Whitehorse, YK
YIA IV8
Email heatherbennetts@hotmail.com

## Regulatory Bodies

### Alberta

The Health Disciplines Board
Alberta Health and Wellness
PO Box 1360, Station Main
Edmonton, AB
T5J 2N3
Tel (780) 427-1432
Fax (780) 422-0102
Email ahinform@health.gov.ab.ca

### British Columbia

College of Midwives of British Columbia
Room F502, 4200 Oak Street
Vancouver, BC
V6H 3N1
Tel (604) 875-3580
Fax (604) 875-3581
Email admin@cmbc.bc.ca

### Manitoba

College of Midwives of Manitoba
235 – 500 Portage Avenue
Winnipeg, MB
R3C 3X1
Tel (204) 783-4520
Fax (204) 779-1490
Web www.midwives.mb.ca
Email admin@midwives.mb.ca

### Newfoundland

Health and Community Services,
   St. John's Region
P.O. Box 13122, Station A
St. John's, NF
A1B 4A4
Tel (709) 738-4800
Web www.commhealth.nf.ca
Email info@hcssjr.nf.ca

### Ontario

College of Midwives of Ontario
2195 Yonge Street, 4th Floor
Toronto, ON
M4S 2B2
Tel (416) 327-0874
Web www.cmo.on.ca
Email admin@cmo.on.ca

### Quebec

L'Ordre des Sages-Femmes du Québec
430, rue Ste-Hélène, bureau 301
Montréal, PQ
H2Y 2K7
Tel (514) 286-1313
Email ordresagesfemmes@qc.aira.com

## Midwifery Education Programs

Midwifery Education Program –
   Laurentian University
Office of Admissions
935 Ramsey Lake Road
Sudbury, ON
P3E 2C6
Tel (705) 675-1151
   1-800-461-4030.
Web www.laurentian.ca
Email liaison@laurentian.ca
         admissions@laurentian.ca

Midwifery Education Program –
   McMaster University
Admissions Coordinator
c/o St. Joseph's Healthcare
Fontbonne Building, 6th Floor
50 Charlton Street East
Hamilton, ON
L8N 4A6
Tel (905) 522-1155 x 5273
Tel (905) 521-6014
Web www.fhs.mcmaster.ca/midwifery

Midwifery Education Programme –
    Ryerson University
Office of Admissions
350 Victoria Street
Toronto, ON
M5B 2K3
Tel (416) 979-5027
    (416) 979-5036
Web www.ryerson.ca/programs/midwifery/html

Midwifery Education Program –
    University of British Columbia
2329 West Mall
Vancouver, BC
V6T 1Z4
Tel (604) 822-2211
Web www.midwifery.ubc.ca

L'Université du Québec à Trois-Rivières
Secretariat du programme sage-femme
3351, boulevard des Forges
Casier Postal 500
Trois Rivières, PQ
G9A 5H7
Tel (819) 376-5011
Fax (819) 376-5012
Web www.ugtr.uquebec.ca

Association for Safe Alternatives in Childbirth
    (ASAC) and *Birth Issues* magazine
Main Post Office Box 1197
Edmonton, AB
T5J 2M4
Tel (780) 425-7993
Fax (780) 497-7576
Web www.asac.ab.ca
Email info@asac.ab.ca

Midwifery Coalition of Nova Scotia
PO Box 33028
Halifax, NS
B3L 4T6
Tel (902) 429-5112
Web www.mcns.chebucto.org/index.htm
Email cjberry@netcom.ca

Groupe Maman
4985, Dornal
Montréal, PQ
H3W 1W1
Tel/Fax (514) 738-4145
Web http://pages.infinit.net/matilda/maman

## Consumer Advocacy Groups

The Midwifery Option
Tel (416) 533-3684
Fax (416) 533-1659
Web www.midwiferyoption.ca
Email info@midwiferyoption.ca

Birth Unlimited and *Birthing* magazine
#C, 3517 – 18 Street SW
Calgary, AB
T2T 4T9
Tel (403) 237-8839
Fax (403) 262-4210
Web www.birthunlimited.ca
Email capsac@telusplanet.net

# Index

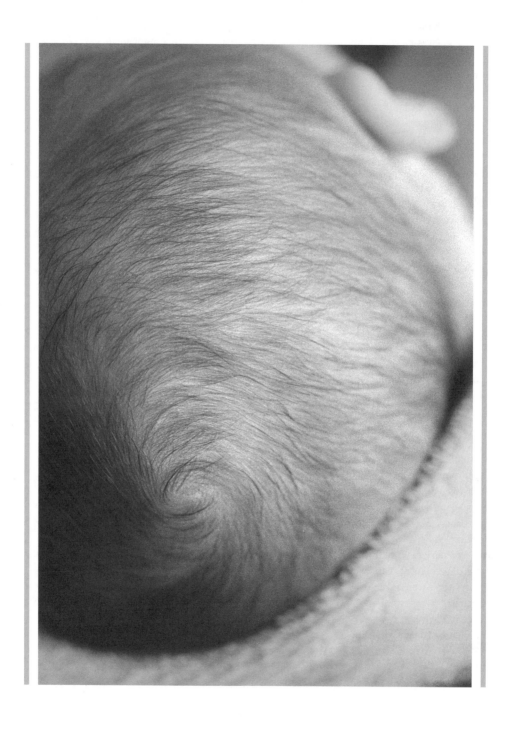